Colposcopy and Treatment of Cervical Intraepithelial Neoplasia:

A Beginners' Manual

INTERNATIONAL AGENCY FOR RESEARCH ON CANCER

The International Agency for Research on Cancer (IARC) was established in 1965 by the World Health Assembly, as an independently financed organization within the framework of the World Health Organization. The headquarters of the Agency are at Lyon, France.

The Agency conducts a programme of research concentrating particularly on the epidemiology of cancer and the study of potential carcinogens in the human environment. Its field studies are supplemented by biological and chemical research carried out in the Agency's laboratories in Lyon, and, through collaborative research agreements, in national research institutions in many countries. The Agency also conducts a programme for the education and training of personnel for cancer research.

The publications of the Agency are intended to contribute to the dissemination of authoritative information on different aspects of cancer research. Information about IARC publications and how to order them is available via the Internet at: **http://www.iarc.fr/**

World Health Organization - International Agency for Research on Cancer (IARC)

World Health Organization Regional Office for Africa (AFRO)

Program for Appropriate Technology in Health (PATH)

International Union Against Cancer (UICC)

International Network for Cancer Treatment and Research (INCTR)

Colposcopy and Treatment of Cervical Intraepithelial Neoplasia:
A Beginners' Manual

John W. Sellors, M.D.
Program for Appropriate Technology in Health
Seattle, Washington, United States

R. Sankaranarayanan, M.D.
International Agency for Research on Cancer
Lyon, France

This publication was funded by a UICC ICRETT Fellowship
and by the Bill & Melinda Gates Foundation
through the Alliance for Cervical Cancer Prevention.

International Agency for Research on Cancer
Lyon, 2003

Published by the International Agency for Research on Cancer,
150 cours Albert Thomas, 69372 Lyon cédex 08, France

© International Agency for Research on Cancer, 2003
Reprinted 2003

Distributed by IARCPress (fax: +33 04 72 73 83 02; E-mail: press@iarc.fr)
and by the World Health Organization Distribution and Sales, CH-1211 Geneva 27 (fax: +41 22 791 4857).

IARC Library Cataloguing in Publication Data

Sellors, John W.
    Colposcopy and treatment of cervical intraepithelial neoplasia : a beginners' manual / John W. Sellors,
R. Sankaranarayanan.

    1.Cervical intraepithelial neoplasia   2.Colposcopy   I. Sankaranarayanan, R.   II.Title

    ISBN   92 832 0412 3 (NLM Classification: QZ 365)

Design and layout by: M J Webb Associates • Newmarket • England

Printed in France

Contents

Foreword vii

Acknowledgements ix

Preface xi

1   An introduction to the anatomy of the uterine cervix 1

2   An introduction to cervical intraepithelial neoplasia (CIN) 13

3   An introduction to invasive cancer of the uterine cervix 21

4   An introduction to colposcopy: indications for colposcopy, ... 29
    instrumentation, principles, and documentation of results

5   The colposcopic examination step-by-step 37

6   Colposcopic appearance of the normal cervix 45

7   Colposcopic assessment of cervical intraepithelial neoplasia 55

8   Colposcopic diagnosis of preclinical invasive carcinoma of the cervix 69
    and glandular neoplasia

9   Inflammatory lesions of the cervix 79

10 Avoiding errors in the colposcopic assessment of the cervix and 85
    colposcopic provisional diagnosis

11   Management that provides continuity of care for women **89**

12   Treatment of cervical intraepithelial neoplasia by cryotherapy **95**

13   Treatment of cervical intraepithelial neoplasia by loop electrosurgical **103**
       excision procedure (LEEP)

14   Decontamination, cleaning, high-level disinfection and sterilisation of **113**
       instruments used during the diagnosis and treatment of cervical neoplasia

       References **117**

       Suggestions for further reading **120**

       Appendices

       1   Example of a colposcopy record **121**

       2   Example of a consent form **123**

       3   Preparation of 5% acetic acid, Lugol's iodine solution, ...   **125**
                  and Monsel's paste

       4   Colposcopic terminology **127**

       5   The modified Reid colposcopic index (RCI) **128**

       Index **131**

Foreword

Women in many developing countries in sub-Saharan Africa, south and south-east Asia, central and south America have a high risk of cervical cancer, and detection programmes and efficient screening programmes are largely lacking. The facilities, service delivery systems and expertise needed for detection and treatment of both cervical precancerous lesions and invasive cancers in many high-risk developing countries are very deficient. Thus, planned investments in health-care infrastructure and in equipping health care providers with skills in cervical cancer prevention are important components of global cervical cancer control initiatives.

Colposcopy is a diagnostic method useful for the diagnosis and evaluation of cervical intraepithelial neoplasia and preclinical invasive cancer. It allows magnified visualization of the site where cervical carcinogenesis occurs. It enables taking directed biopsy and in delineating the extent of lesions on the cervix in screen-positive women, thus avoiding conization. It also helps in directing treatments such as cryotherapy and loop electrosurgical excision procedure for cervical intraepithelial neoplasia. Colposcopy is not widely available and not widely practised in many developing countries where a high incidence of cervical cancer is observed. Similarly, skills and facilities for cryotherapy and loop electrosurgical excision procedure, the two appropriate treatment methods for cervical intraepithelial neoplasia in low-resource settings discussed in this manual, are extremely deficient in many developing countries at high risk for cervical cancer.

This introductory manual is intended to simplify the learning of colposcopy and treatment of cervical intraepithelial neoplasia with cryotherapy and loop electrosurgical excision procedure so as to allow dissemination of the skills in low-resource settings. The first draft of the manual was written as a result of an ICRETT fellowship, offered by the International Union Against Cancer (UICC). Subsequently, the manual was used in a number of training courses in developing countries to train health care personnel in colposcopy and treatment of cervical intraepithelial neoplasia, in the context of specific research and demonstration projects in early detection and prevention of cervical cancer. The feedback from those courses, and from users and the reviewers of draft versions of this manual, has been helpful to further improve the contents.

It is hoped that this manual will find a range of uses, as a resource for short teaching courses for health-care personnel, as a teaching, as well as a learning, aid for medical and nursing students, medical practitioners, as a field manual in screening programmes or even as a self-learning tool. Availability of simplified learning resources, training mechanisms and trained providers in cervical cancer prevention may help to overcome some of the technical challenges and may prepare the ground for implementing such services in developing countries. We believe that this manual will help to equip health care providers with the necessary skills in detecting and treating cervical intraepithelial neoplasia, thereby preventing invasive cervical cancer in many women world-wide.

P. Kleihues, M.D.
Director, IARC

C. Elias, M.D.
President, PATH

Acknowledgements

The authors gratefully acknowledge the following colleagues who readily agreed to review a draft version of this manual, in spite of short notice, and who provided useful suggestions, advice for revision and encouragement. The manual has greatly benefited from their input. Nevertheless, the sole responsibility for the content remains the authors' and we wish to impress the fact that the recommendations in this manual have been made based on what we think is feasible and effective in low-resource settings:

Dr Parthasarathy Basu, Gynaecological Oncology, Chittaranjan National Cancer Institute, S.P. Mukherjee Road, Calcutta, India

Dr Jerome Belinson, Gynecologic Oncology, The Cleveland Clinic Foundation, Cleveland, Ohio, USA.

Dr Neerja Bhatla, Associate Professor of Obstetrics & Gynaecology, All India Institute of Medical Sciences, New Delhi, India

Dr Paul D. Blumenthal, Director, Contraceptive Research and Programs, Johns Hopkins Bayview Medical Center, Associate Professor, Department of Gynaecology and Obstetrics, Johns Hopkins University, Baltimore, MD, USA

Dr Nagindra Das, Department of Gynaecological Oncolgy, Northern Gynaecology Oncology Centre, Gateshead, Tyne & Wear, England

Dr Lynette Denny, Department of Obstetrics & Gynaecology, Faculty of Health Sciences, Cape Town, South Africa

Dr Amadou Dolo, Chef de Service Gynécologie-Obstetrique, Hôpital Gabriel Touré, Bamako, Mali

Dr Laurie Elit, Hamilton Regional Cancer Centre, Hamilton, Ontario, Canada

Dr Alex Ferenczy, Professor of Pathology and Obstetrics and Gynaecology, The Sir Mortimer B. Davis Jewish General Hospital, Montreal, Canada

Dr Daron Ferris, Director, Student Health Service, Associate Professor, Department of Family Medicine Medical College of Georgia, Student Health Center, Augusta, GA, USA

Dr Bernard Fontanière, Professor of Cytology, Centre Leon Berard, Lyon, France

Dr Silvia Franceschi, Chief of the Unit of Field Intervention Studies, IARC, Lyon, France

Dr L. Frappart, Laboratoire d'Anatomie et de Cytologie Pathologiques, Hôpital Edouard Herriot, Lyon, France

Dr K. Geethanjali Amin, Department of Preventive Oncology, Tata Memorial Center, Mumbai, India

Dr José Jeronimo Guibovich, Ginecologia Oncologia, Patalogia Mamaria, Colposcopia, Instituto de Enfermedades Neoplasicas, Lima, Peru

Dr Robert D. Hilgers, Executive Director, International Gynecologic Cancer Society, Louisville KY, USA

Dr Martha Jacob, EngenderHealth, New York, NY, USA

Dr Namory Keita, Chef de Service de Gynécologie - Obstétrique, Université de Conakry, CHU Donka, Conakry, Guinée

Dr Peter H. Kilmarx, U.S.Centers for Disease Control and Prevention, USA

Dr Suphannee Koonsaeng, Gynecologic Oncology Unit, National Cancer Institute, Bangkok, Thailand

Dr R. Lambert, Unit of Descriptive Epidemiology, IARC, Lyon, France

Dr Jean Liaras, Caluire, Lyon, France

Dr Pisake Lumbiganon, Professor and Chairman, Department of Obstetrics & Gynaecology, Faculty of Medicine, Khon Kaen University, Khon Kaen, Thailand

Dr Monique Marien, Department of Obstetrics & Gynaecology, Hôpital Edouard Herriot, Lyon, France

Dr Patrice Mathevet, Department of Obstetrics & Gynaecology, Hôpital Edouard Herriot, Lyon, France

Dr Paulo Naud, Co-ordinator, Programme on Detection of Precursor Lesions of Cervical Cancer and HPV Infection, Porte Alegre, RS - Brazil

Dr B.M. Nene, Chairman, Tata Memorial Centre Rural Cancer Project, Nargis Dutt Memorial Cancer Hospital, Agalgaon Road, Barshi District – Solapur, Maharashtra, India

Dr D. Maxwell Parkin, Chief of the Unit of Descriptive Epidemiology, IARC, Lyon, France

Dr R. Rajeswarkar, Tata Memorial Centre Rural Cancer Project, Nargis Dutt Memorial Cancer Hospital, Agalgaon Road, Barshi District – Solapur, Maharashtra, India

Dr R. Rajkumar, Christian Fellowship Community Health Centre, Ambillikai, Dindigul District, Tamil Nadu, India

Dr Ralph Richart, Obstetrical and Gynaecological Pathology, College of Physicians and Surgeons, Colombia University, New York, NY, USA

Dr Jose Antonio Ruiz Moreno, Department of Obstetrics and Gynaecology, Central Military Hospital, Mexico City, Mexico

Dr Carlos L. Santos, Chairman, Gynecologic Oncology Department, Insituto de Enfermedades Neoplasicas, Lima, Peru

Dr Paul Sebastian, Chief of Surgical Oncology, Regional Cancer Centre, Trivandrum, India

Dr Aarati Shah, Director, Bhaktapur Cancer Care Centre, Bhaktapur, Nepal

Dr Thara Somanathan, Assistant Professor of Pathology, Regional Cancer Centre, Trivandrum, India

Mr Pat Soutter, Reader in Gynaecological Oncology, Hammersmith & Queen Charlotte's Hospital, London, England

Dr Sudha S. Sundar, John Radcliffe Hospital, Oxford, England

Dr Ramani Wesley, Associate Professor of Community Oncology, Regional Cancer Center, Medical College Campus, Trivandrum, Kerala State, India

Dr Thomas C. Wright Jr, Associate Professor of Pathology, Director, Obstetrical and Gynaecological Pathology, College of Physicians and Surgeons, Colombia University, New York, NY, USA

Finally, the authors are very grateful to all the students of the training courses where this manual was used, for their helpful suggestions.

The authors are grateful to the following colleagues for permission to reproduce photographs and diagrams:

Mr Pat Soutter, Reader in Gynaecological Oncology, Hammersmith Hospitals NHS Trust, London, United Kingdom, for Figure 1.10 b (From: Soutter P. *Practical Colposcopy.* Oxford University Press, Oxford, 1993).

Dr Alex Ferenczy, Professor of Pathology and Obstetrics and Gynaecology, The Sir Mortimer B. Davis Jewish General Hospital, Montreal (Quebec), Canada, for Figures 13.4, 13.6 and 13.7 (From: Thomas C. Wright, Ralph M. Richart, Alex Ferenczy. *Electrosurgery for HPV-related Diseases of the Lower Genital Tract.* Arthur and BioVision, Inc, New City, New York, USA and Anjou, Quebec, Canada, 1992).

Ms Marylene Riopille, Publisher, Biomedical Communications, 3609 Cason Street, Houston, TX 77005, USA, for Figures 6.2, 7.2a, 8.5 (From: V. Cecil Wright, Gordon M. Lickrish, R. Michael Shier. *Basic and Advanced Colposcopy.* Second Edition, Biomedical Communications, Houston, 1995).

Mr J.A. Jordan, President of the European Federation of Colposcopy & Pathology of the Lower Genital Tract, Consultant Gynaecologist, Birmingham Women's Hospital, Birmingham, UK for Figures 1.4, 6.2, 7.3, (From: M.C. Anderson, J.A. Jordan, A.R. Morse, F. Sharp, A Stafl. *Integrated Colposcopy.* Second Edition. Chapman Hall Medical, London and New York. 1996).

Dr Paul Blumenthal, Director, Contraceptive Research and Programs, Johns Hopkins Bayview Medical Center, Baltimore, USA for Figure 12.5 (From: N. McIntosh, P. Blumenthal, A. Blouse. *Cervical Cancer Prevention guidelines for low-resource settings.* JHPIEGO Corporation, Baltimore, Global Draft 2000).

The authors are also very much indebted to the following colleagues for their valuable, tireless, patient and perseverant contribution in the preparation of this manual, without which we would have found the task much more difficult:

Dr John Cheney, IARC, Lyon, France, who undertook the task of editing this manual;

Mrs Evelyn Bayle, IARC, Lyon, France, who undertook the preliminary editing and typing of the several draft versions of this manual;

Ms Krittika Pitaksaringkarn, IARC, Lyon, France, who helped in the imaging of the diagrams;

Mrs Lakshmi Sankaranarayanan, Lyon, France, who helped with the line drawings of illustrations.

Preface

Health care providers have observed a high incidence of cervical cancer in many developing countries in Africa, Asia, and Central and South America, and in the absence of organized early-detection programmes the mortality rates from this disease remain high. The extremely limited health-care infrastructure available in many of these countries contributes to a compelling need to build a capacity to identify cervical neoplasia in early, preventable stages, preferably even before - and not in the wake of - the introduction of early detection programmes in such settings. Colposcopy is generally regarded as a diagnostic test; it is used to assess women who have been identified to have cervical abnormalities on various screening tests.

This introductory manual for gynaecologists, pathologists, general practitioners, and nurses is intended to provide information on the principles of colposcopy and the basic skills needed to colposcopically assess cervical intraepithelial neoplasia and to provide basic treatment. Interested health professionals are expected to subsequently continue to improve their skills by undertaking a basic course of theoretical and practical training, and by referring to standard textbooks dealing with the subject more extensively. Continuing practical work is vital for acquiring, improving and sustaining necessary skills in the colposcopic diagnosis of cervical neoplasia. This manual is also intended to be a beginner's self-learning resource and as a teaching aid for colposcopy courses for health care personnel, as well as a resource for teaching curricula for medical and nursing students in developing countries. It may also be used as a field manual in routine screening programmes.

A good understanding of the gross and microscopic anatomy of the uterine cervix, infective and inflammatory conditions of the cervix and the vagina, histology and the natural history of cervical neoplasia is absolutely essential for a correct interpretation of colposcopic findings and colposcopic diagnosis of cervical neoplasia. These aspects are dealt with in detail in this manual, and should be well studied in conjunction with other chapters dealing with colposcopic techniques and features of cervical neoplasia and their treatment.

Generally speaking, colposcopy should not be practised unless the provider has had an opportunity to spend some time with an experienced colposcopist. Unfortunately, this is extremely difficult to arrange in most of the developing world, where the disease incidence is high (particularly in sub-Saharan Africa) and both access to such training and to a colposcope is rarely available. For instance, quite apart from colposcopy training, no colposcopy service itself is available in whole regions of Africa and Asia and Latin America. Realistically, the basic colposcopist in such situations is a self-trained health-care provider who knows how to examine the cervix, what to look for, how to make a diagnosis, and how to treat a woman with simple ablative or excisional methods. We emphasize, however, that an instructor should be available for the on-site training of new colposcopists. The limitations and far-reaching implications of incomplete understanding of cervical disease and inadequate expertise should be well appreciated by potential practitioners.

Draft versions of this manual have been used in more than 20 courses on colposcopy and management of cervical precancers conducted in Angola, Congo (Brazzaville), Guinea, Kenya, India, Mali, Mauritania, Laos and Tanzania. More than 120 doctors and nurses have been trained and initiated in colposcopy in the context of the cervical cancer prevention research initiatives in these countries as well as in other countries such as Burkina Faso, Cape Verde, Equatorial Guinea, Mozambique, Nepal, Niger, Sao Tome and Uganda. Feedback from the participants and teaching faculty of these courses has been particularly useful in revising the draft versions of the manual. The illustrations used in this manual have also largely been drawn from the above-mentioned country projects.

The resource constraints for health-care systems in many developing countries are substantial, with practical challenges on how colposcopy and treatment of early cervical neoplasia can be integrated into and delivered through these health services. Awareness of these limitations will pave the way to establishing, integrating, and maintaining such services within the health-care infrastructure of developing countries. We hope that this manual will help the learner, given access to a colposcope, to start performing colposcopy and recognizing lesions, and in effectively treating them with cryotherapy or loop electrosurgical excision procedure (LEEP). We believe that, in due course, it will catalyse and contribute to the initiation and dissemination of preventive services for cervical cancer in low-resource regions and countries.

John W. Sellors M.D.
R. Sankaranarayanan M.D.

Chapter 1

An introduction to the anatomy of the uterine cervix

- The cervix, the lower fibromuscular portion of the uterus, measures 3-4 cm in length and 2.5 cm in diameter; however, it varies in size and shape depending on age, parity and menstrual status of the woman.

- Ectocervix is the most readily visible portion of the cervix; endocervix is largely invisible and lies proximal to the external os.

- Ectocervix is covered by a pink stratified squamous epithelium, consisting of multiple layers of cells and a reddish columnar epithelium consisting of a single layer of cells lines the endocervix. The intermediate and superficial cell layers of the squamous epithelium contain glycogen.

- The location of squamocolumnar junction in relation to the external os varies depending upon age, menstrual status, and other factors such as pregnancy and oral contraceptive use.

- Ectropion refers to the eversion of the columnar epithelium onto the ectocervix, when the cervix grows rapidly and enlarges under the influence of estrogen, after menarche and during pregnancy.

- Squamous metaplasia in the cervix refers to the physiological replacement of the everted columnar epithelium on the ectocervix by a newly formed squamous epithelium from the subcolumnar reserve cells.

- The region of the cervix where squamous metaplasia occurs is referred to as the transformation zone.

- Identifying the transformation zone is of great importance in colposcopy, as almost all manifestations of cervical carcinogenesis occur in this zone.

A thorough understanding of the anatomy and physiology of the cervix is absolutely essential for effective colposcopic practice. This chapter deals with the gross and microscopic anatomy of the uterine cervix and the physiology of the transformation zone. The cervix is the lower fibromuscular portion of the uterus. It is cylindrical or conical in shape, and measures 3 to 4 cm in length, and 2.5 cm in diameter. It is supported by the cardinal and uterosacral ligaments, which stretch between the lateral and posterior portions of the cervix and the walls of the bony pelvis. The lower half of the cervix, called the portio vaginalis, protrudes into the vagina through its anterior wall, and the upper half remains above the vagina (Figure 1.1). The portio vaginalis opens into the vagina through an orifice called the external os.

The cervix varies in size and shape depending on the woman's age, parity and hormonal status. In parous women, it is bulky and the external os appears as a wide, gaping, transverse slit. In nulliparous women, the external os resembles a small circular opening in the centre of the cervix. The supravaginal portion meets with the muscular body of the uterus at the internal cervical os. The portion of the cervix lying exterior to the external os is called the ectocervix. This is the portion of the cervix that is

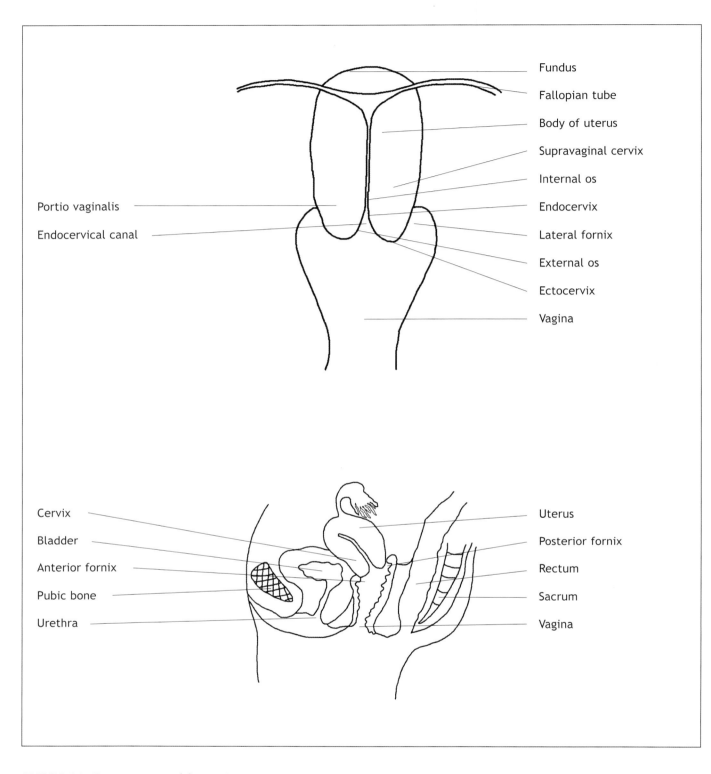

FIGURE 1.1: Gross anatomy of the uterine cervix

readily visible on speculum examination. The portion proximal to the external os is called the endocervix and the external os needs to be stretched or dilated to view this portion of the cervix. The endocervical canal, which traverses the endocervix, connects the uterine cavity with the vagina and extends from the internal to the external os, where it opens into the vagina. It varies in length and width depending on the woman's age and hormonal status. It is widest in women in the reproductive age group, when it measures 6-8 mm in width.

The space surrounding the cervix in the vaginal cavity is called the vaginal fornix. The part of the fornix between the cervix and the lateral vaginal walls is called the lateral fornix; the portions between the anterior and posterior walls of the vagina and the cervix are termed the anterior and posterior fornix, respectively.

The stroma of the cervix is composed of dense, fibro-muscular tissue through which vascular, lymphatic and nerve supplies to the cervix pass and form a complex plexus. The arterial supply of the cervix is derived from internal iliac arteries through the cervical and vaginal branches of the uterine arteries. The cervical branches of the uterine arteries descend in the lateral aspects of the cervix at 3 and 9 o'clock positions. The veins of the cervix run parallel to the arteries and drain into the hypogastric venous plexus. The lymphatic vessels from the cervix drain into the common, external and internal iliac nodes, obturator and the parametrial nodes. The nerve supply to the cervix is derived from the hypogastric plexus. The endocervix has extensive sensory nerve endings, while there are very few in the ectocervix. Hence, procedures such as biopsy, electrocoagulation and cryotherapy are well tolerated in most women without local anaesthesia. Since sympathetic and parasympathetic fibres are also abundant in the endocervix, dilatation and curettage of the endocervix may occasionally lead to a vasovagal reaction.

The cervix is covered by both stratified non-keratinizing squamous and columnar epithelium. These two types of epithelium meet at the squamocolumnar junction.

Stratified non-keratinizing squamous epithelium

Normally, a large area of ectocervix is covered by a stratified, non-keratinizing, glycogen-containing squamous epithelium. It is opaque, has multiple (15-20) layers of cells (Figure 1.2) and is pale pink in colour. This epithelium may be native to the site formed during embryonic life, which is called the native or original squamous epithelium, or it may have been newly formed as metaplastic squamous epithelium in early adult life. In premenopausal women, the original squamous epithelium is pinkish in colour, whereas the newly formed metaplastic squamous epithelium looks somewhat pinkish-white on visual examination.

The histological architecture of the squamous epithelium of the cervix reveals, at the bottom, a single layer of round basal cells with a large dark-staining nuclei and little cytoplasm, attached to the basement membrane (Figure 1.2). The basement membrane separates the epithelium from the underlying stroma. The epithelial-stromal junction is usually straight. Sometimes it is slightly undulating with short projections of stroma at regular intervals. These stromal projections are called papillae. The parts of the epithelium between the papillae are called rete pegs.

The basal cells divide and mature to form the next few layers of cells called parabasal cells, which also have relatively large dark-staining nuclei and greenish-blue basophilic cytoplasm. Further

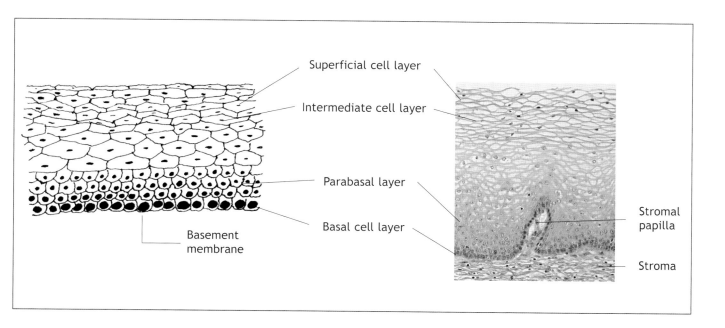

Superficial cell layer

Intermediate cell layer

Parabasal layer

Basal cell layer

Basement membrane

Stromal papilla

Stroma

FIGURE 1.2: Stratified squamous epithelium (x 20)

differentiation and maturation of these cells leads to the intermediate layers of polygonal cells with abundant cytoplasm and small round nuclei. These cells form a basket-weave pattern. With further maturation, the large and markedly flattened cells with small, dense, pyknotic nuclei and transparent cytoplasm of the superficial layers are formed. Overall, from the basal to the superficial layer, these cells undergo an increase in size and a reduction of nuclear size.

The intermediate and superficial layer cells contain abundant glycogen in their cytoplasm, which stains mahogany brown or black after application of Lugol's iodine and magenta with periodic acid-Schiff stain in histological sections. Glycogenation of the intermediate and superficial layers is a sign of normal maturation and development of the squamous epithelium. Abnormal or altered maturation is characterized by a lack of glycogen production.

The maturation of the squamous epithelium of the cervix is dependent on estrogen, the female hormone. If estrogen is lacking, full maturation and glycogenation does not take place. Hence, after menopause, the cells do not mature beyond the parabasal layer and do not accumulate as multiple layers of flat cells. Consequently, the epithelium becomes thin and atrophic. On visual examination, it appears pale, with subepithelial petechial haemorrhagic spots, as it is easily prone to trauma.

Columnar epithelium

The endocervical canal is lined by the columnar epithelium (sometimes referred to as glandular epithelium). It is composed of a single layer of tall cells with dark-staining nuclei close to the basement membrane (Figure 1.3). Because of its single layer of cells, it is much shorter in height than the stratified squamous epithelium of the cervix. On visual

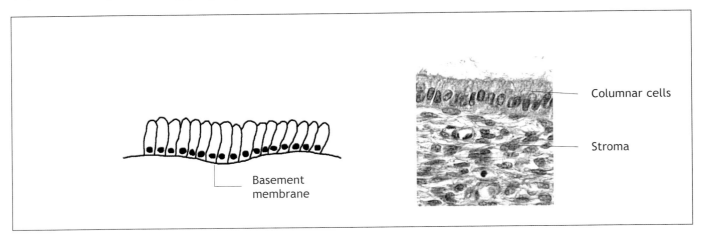

FIGURE 1.3: Columnar epithelium (x 40)

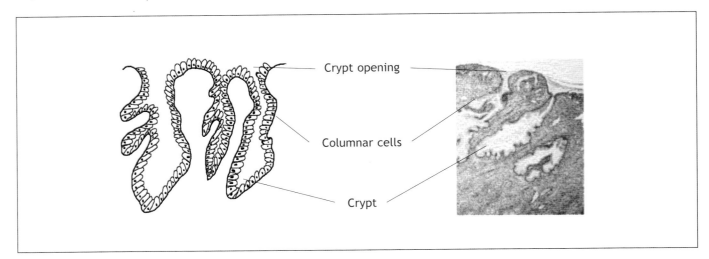

FIGURE 1.4: Crypts of columnar epithelium (x 10)

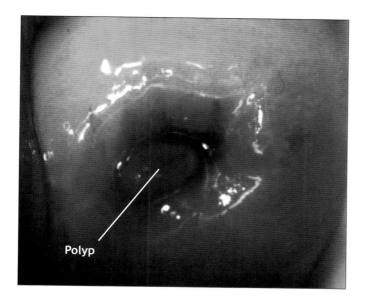

FIGURE 1.5: Cervical polyp

examination, it appears reddish in colour because the thin single cell layer allows the coloration of the underlying vasculature in the stroma to be seen more easily. At its distal or upper limit, it merges with the endometrial epithelium in the lower part of the body of the uterus. At its proximal or lower limit, it meets with the squamous epithelium at the squamocolumnar junction. It covers a variable extent of the ectocervix, depending upon the woman's age, reproductive, hormonal and menopausal status.

The columnar epithelium does not form a flattened surface in the cervical canal, but is thrown into multiple longitudinal folds protruding into the lumen of the canal, giving rise to papillary projections. It forms several invaginations into the substance of the cervical stroma, resulting in the formation of endocervical

crypts (sometimes referred to as endocervical glands) (Figure 1.4). The crypts may traverse as far as 5-8 mm from the surface of the cervix. This complex architecture, consisting of mucosal folds and crypts, gives the columnar epithelium a grainy appearance on visual inspection.

A localized overgrowth of the endocervical columnar epithelium may occasionally be visible as a reddish mass protruding from the external os on visual examination of the cervix. This is called a cervical polyp (Figure 1.5). It usually begins as a localized enlargement of a single columnar papilla and appears as a mass as it enlarges. It is composed of a core of endocervical stroma lined by the columnar epithelium with underlying crypts. Occasionally, multiple polyps may arise from the columnar epithelium.

Glycogenation and mitoses are absent in the columnar epithelium. Because of the lack of intracytoplasmic glycogen, the columnar epithelium does not change colour after the application of Lugol's iodine or remains slightly discoloured with a thin film of iodine solution.

Squamocolumnar junction

The squamocolumnar junction (Figures 1.6 and 1.7) appears as a sharp line with a step, due to the difference in the height of the squamous and columnar epithelium. The location of the squamocolumnar junction in relation to the external os is variable over a woman's lifetime and depends upon factors such as age, hormonal status, birth trauma, oral contraceptive use and certain physiological conditions such as pregnancy (Figures 1.6 and 1.7).

The squamocolumnar junction visible during childhood, perimenarche, after puberty and early

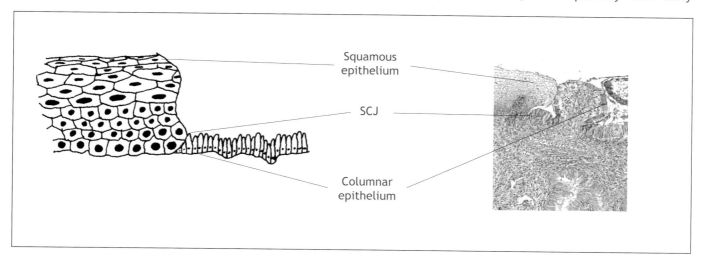

FIGURE 1.6: Squamocolumnar junction (SCJ) (x 10)

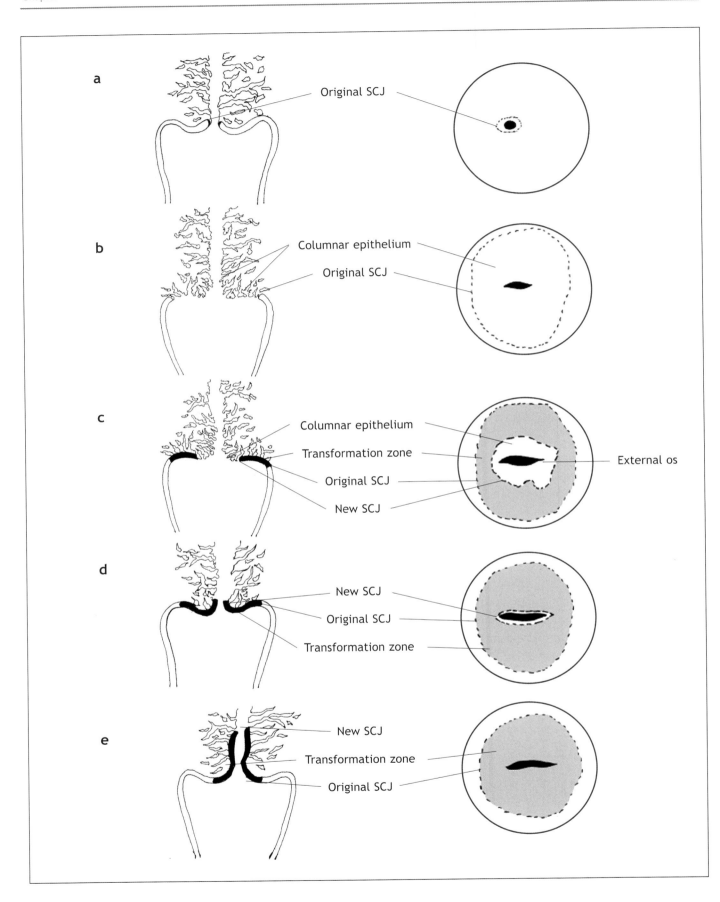

FIGURE 1.7: Location of the squamocolumnar junction (SCJ) and transformation zone; (a) before menarche; (b) after puberty and at early reproductive age; (c) in a woman in her 30s; (d) in a perimenopausal woman; (e) in a postmenopausal woman

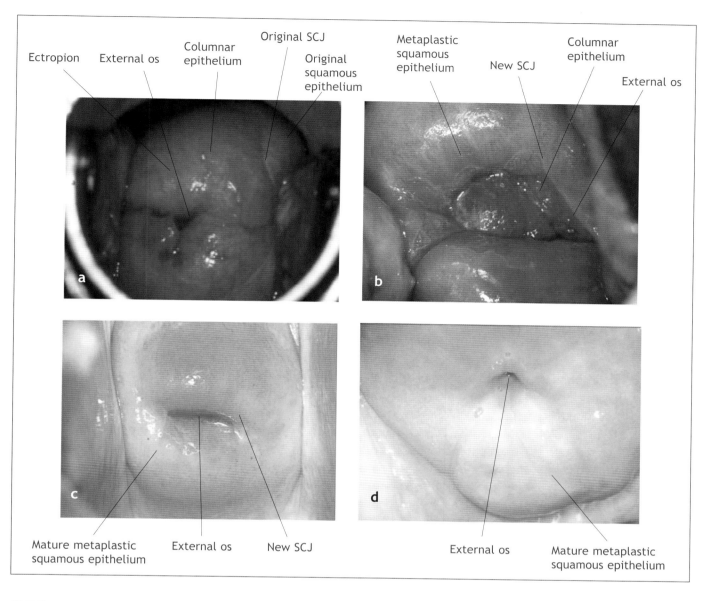

Ectropion   External os   Columnar epithelium   Original SCJ   Original squamous epithelium

Metaplastic squamous epithelium   New SCJ   Columnar epithelium   External os

Mature metaplastic squamous epithelium   External os   New SCJ

External os   Mature metaplastic squamous epithelium

FIGURE 1.8: Location of squamocolumnar junction (SCJ)

(a)   Original squamocolumnar junction (SCJ) in a young woman in the early reproductive age group. The SCJ is located far away from the external os. Note the presence of everted columnar epithelium occupying a large portion of the ectocervix producing ectropion

(b)   The new SCJ has moved much closer to the external os in a woman in her 30s. The SCJ is visible as a distinct white line after the application of 5% acetic acid due to the presence of immature squamous metaplastic epithelium adjacent to the new SCJ

(c)   The new SCJ is at the external os in a perimenopausal woman

(d)   The new SCJ is not visible and has receded into the endocervix in a postmenopausal woman. Mature metaplastic squamous epithelium occupies most of the ectocervix

reproductive period is referred to as the original squamocolumnar junction, as this represents the junction between the columnar epithelium and the 'original' squamous epithelium laid down during embryogenesis and intrauterine life. During childhood and perimenarche, the original squamocolumnar junction is located at, or very close to, the external os (Figure 1.7a). After puberty and during the

reproductive period, the female genital organs grow under the influence of estrogen. Thus, the cervix swells and enlarges and the endocervical canal elongates. This leads to the eversion of the columnar epithelium of the lower part of the endocervical canal on to the ectocervix (Figure 1.7b). This condition is called ectropion or ectopy, which is visible as a strikingly reddish-looking ectocervix on visual inspection

(Figure 1.8a). It is sometimes called 'erosion' or 'ulcer', which are misnomers and should not be used to denote this condition. Thus the original squamocolumnar junction is located on the ectocervix, far away from the external os (Figures 1.7b and 1.8a). Ectropion becomes much more pronounced during pregnancy.

The buffer action of the mucus covering the columnar cells is interfered with when the everted columnar epithelium in ectropion is exposed to the acidic vaginal environment. This leads to the destruction and eventual replacement of the columnar epithelium by the newly formed metaplastic squamous epithelium. Metaplasia refers to the change or replacement of one type of epithelium by another.

The metaplastic process mostly starts at the original squamocolumnar junction and proceeds centripetally towards the external os through the reproductive period to perimenopause. Thus, a new squamocolumnar junction is formed between the newly formed metaplastic squamous epithelium and the columnar epithelium remaining everted onto the ectocervix (Figures 1.7c, 1.8b). As the woman passes from the reproductive to the perimenopausal age group, the location of the new squamocolumnar junction progressively moves on the ectocervix towards the external os (Figures 1.7c, 1.7d, 1.7e and 1.8). Hence, it is located at variable distances from the external os, as a result of the progressive formation of the new metaplastic squamous epithelium in the exposed areas of the columnar epithelium in the ectocervix. From the perimenopausal period and after the onset of menopause, the cervix shrinks due the lack of estrogen, and consequently, the movement of the new squamocolumnar junction towards the external os and into the endocervical canal is accelerated (Figures 1.7d and 1.8c). In postmenopausal women, the new squamocolumnar junction is often invisible on visual examination (Figures 1.7e and 1.8d).

The new squamocolumnar junction is hereafter simply referred to as squamocolumnar junction in this manual. Reference to the original squamocolumnar junction will be explicitly made as the original squamocolumnar junction.

Ectropion or ectopy

Ectropion or ectopy is defined as the presence of everted endocervical columnar epithelium on the ectocervix. It appears as a large reddish area on the ectocervix surrounding the external os (Figures 1.7b and 1.8a). The eversion of the columnar epithelium is more pronounced on the anterior and posterior lips of the ectocervix and less on the lateral lips. This is a normal, physiological occurrence in a woman's life. Occasionally the columnar epithelium extends into the vaginal fornix. The whole mucosa including the crypts and the supporting stroma is displaced in ectropion. It is the region in which physiological transformation to squamous metaplasia, as well as abnormal transformation in cervical carcinogenesis, occurs.

Squamous metaplasia

The physiological replacement of the everted columnar epithelium by a newly formed squamous epithelium is called squamous metaplasia. The vaginal environment is acidic during the reproductive years and during pregnancy. The acidity is thought to play a role in squamous metaplasia. When the cells are repeatedly destroyed by vaginal acidity in the columnar epithelium in an area of ectropion, they are eventually replaced by a newly formed metaplastic epithelium. The irritation of exposed columnar epithelium by the acidic vaginal environment results in the appearance of sub-columnar reserve cells. These cells proliferate producing a reserve cell hyperplasia and eventually form the metaplastic squamous epithelium.

As already indicated, the metaplastic process requires the appearance of undifferentiated, cuboidal, sub-columnar cells called reserve cells (Figure 1.9a), for the metaplastic squamous epithelium is produced from the multiplication and differentiation of these cells. These eventually lift off the persistent columnar epithelium (Figures 1.9b and 1.9c). The exact origin of the reserve cells is not known, though it is widely believed that it develops from the columnar epithelium, in response to irritation by the vaginal acidity.

The first sign of squamous metaplasia is the appearance and proliferation of reserve cells (Figures 1.9a and 1.9b). This is initially seen as a single layer of small, round cells with darkly staining nuclei, situated very close to the nuclei of columnar cells, which further proliferate to produce a reserve cell hyperplasia (Figure 1.9b). Morphologically, the reserve cells have a similar appearance to the basal cells of the original squamous epithelium, with round nuclei and little cytoplasm. As the metaplastic process progresses, the reserve cells proliferate and differentiate to form a thin, multicellular epithelium of immature squamous cells with no evidence of stratification (Figure 1.9c). The term immature

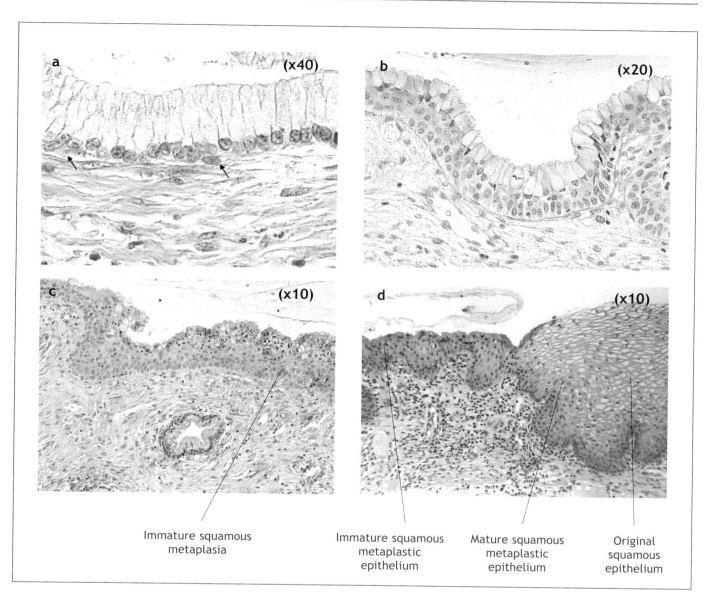

Immature squamous
metaplasia

Immature squamous
metaplastic
epithelium

Mature squamous
metaplastic
epithelium

Original
squamous
epithelium

FIGURE 1.9: Development of squamous metaplastic epithelium

(a) The arrows indicate the appearance of the subcolumnar reserve cells

(b) The reserve cells proliferate to form two layers of reserve cell hyperplasia beneath the overlying layer of columnar epithelium

(c) The reserve cells further proliferate and differentiate to form immature squamous metaplastic epithelium. There is no evidence of glycogen production

(d) Mature squamous metaplastic epithelium is indistinguishable from the original squamous epithelium for all practical purposes

squamous metaplastic epithelium is applied when there is little or no stratification in this thin newly formed metaplastic epithelium. The cells in the immature squamous metaplastic epithelium do not produce glycogen and, hence, do not stain brown or black with Lugol's iodine solution. Groups of mucin-containing columnar cells may be seen embedded in the immature squamous metaplastic epithelium at this stage.

Numerous continuous and/or isolated fields or foci of immature squamous metaplasia may arise at the same time. It has been proposed that the basement membrane of the original columnar epithelium dissolves and is reformed between the proliferating and differentiating reserve cells and the cervical stroma. Squamous metaplasia usually begins at the original squamocolumnar junction at the distal limit of the ectopy, but it may also occur in the columnar epithelium close to this junction or as islands scattered in the exposed columnar epithelium.

As the process continues, the immature metaplastic squamous cells differentiate into mature stratified metaplastic epithelium (Figure 1.9d). For all practical

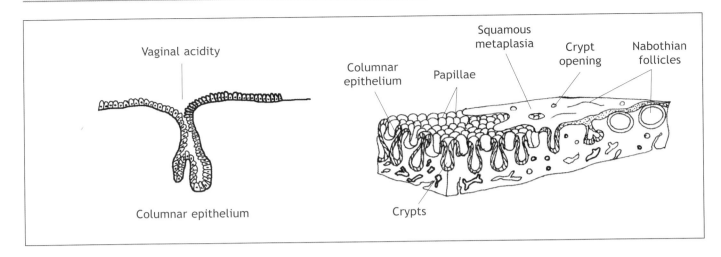

FIGURE 1.10: Squamous metaplastic epithelium covering the crypt openings, leading to the formation of nabothian retention cysts

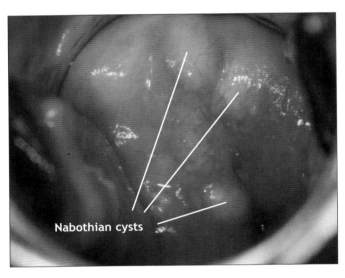

FIGURE 1.11: Multiple nabothian cysts in the mature squamous metaplastic epithelium occupying the ectocervix

purposes, the latter resembles the original stratified squamous epithelium. Some residual columnar cells or vacuoles of mucus are seen in the mature squamous metaplastic epithelium, which contains glycogen from the intermediate cell layer onwards. Thus, it stains brown or black after application of Lugol's iodine. Several cysts, called nabothian cysts (follicles), may be observed in the mature metaplastic squamous epithelium (Figures 1.10 and 1.11). Nabothian cysts are retention cysts that develop as a result of the occlusion of an endocervical crypt opening or outlet by the overlying metaplastic squamous epithelium (Figure 1.10). The buried columnar epithelium continues to secrete mucus, which eventually fills and distends the cyst. The entrapped mucus gives an ivory-white to yellowish hue to the cyst on visual examination (Figure 1.11). The columnar epithelium in the wall of the cyst

is flattened and ultimately destroyed by the pressure of the mucus in it. The outlets of the crypts of columnar epithelium, not yet covered by the metaplastic epithelium, remain as persistent crypt openings. The farthest extent of the metaplastic epithelium onto the ectocervix can be best judged by the location of the crypt opening farthest away from the squamocolumnar junction.

Squamous metaplasia is an irreversible process; the transformed epithelium (now squamous in character) cannot revert to columnar epithelium. The metaplastic process in the cervix is sometimes referred to as indirect metaplasia, as the columnar cells do not transform into squamous cells, but are replaced by the proliferating sub-columnar cuboidal reserve cells. Squamous metaplasia may progress at varying rates in different areas of the same cervix, and hence many areas of widely differing maturity may be seen in the metaplastic squamous epithelium with or without islands of columnar epithelium. The metaplastic epithelium adjacent to the squamocolumnar junction is composed of immature metaplasia, and the mature metaplastic epithelium is found near the original squamocolumnar junction.

Further development of the newly formed immature metaplastic epithelium may take two directions (Figure 1.12). In the vast majority of women, it develops into a mature squamous metaplastic epithelium, which is similar to the normal glycogen-containing original squamous epithelium for all practical purposes. In a very small minority of women, an atypical, dysplastic epithelium may develop. Certain oncogenic human papillomavirus (HPV) types may persistently infect the immature basal squamous metaplastic cells and transform them into atypical

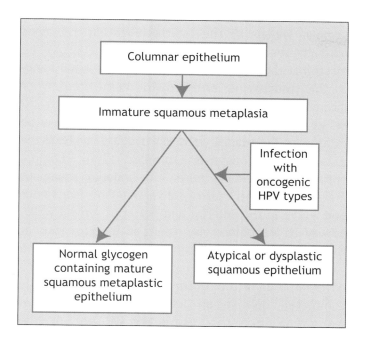

FIGURE 1.12: A schematic diagram of further maturation of immature squamous metaplasia

cells with nuclear and cytoplasmic abnormalities. The uncontrolled proliferation and expansion of these atypical cells may lead to the formation of an abnormal dysplastic epithelium which may regress to normal, persist as dysplasia or progress into invasive cancer after several years.

It is also thought that some metaplasia may occur by in-growth of the squamous epithelium from the squamous epithelium of the ectocervix.

Transformation zone

This region of the cervix where the columnar epithelium has been replaced and/or is being replaced by the new metaplastic squamous epithelium is referred to as the transformation zone. It corresponds to the area of cervix bound by the original squamocolumnar junction at the distal end and proximally by the furthest extent that squamous metaplasia has occurred as defined by the new squamocolumnar junction (Figures 1.7, 1.13 and 1.14).

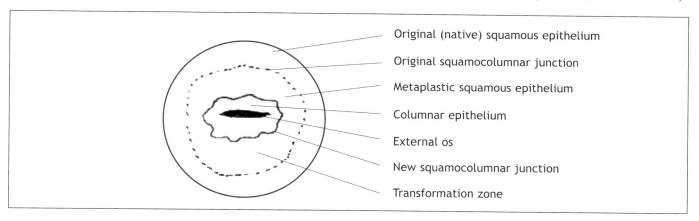

FIGURE 1.13: A schematic diagram of the transformation zone

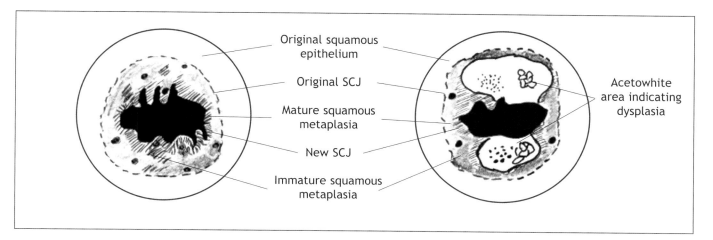

FIGURE 1.14: (a) A schematic diagram of the normal transformation zone; (b) a schematic diagram of the abnormal or atypical transformation zone harbouring dysplasia

11

In premenopausal women, the transformation zone is fully located on the ectocervix. After menopause through old age, the cervix shrinks with the decreasing levels of estrogen. Consequently, the transformation zone may move partially, and later fully, into the cervical canal.

The transformation zone may be described as normal when it is composed of immature and/or mature squamous metaplasia along with intervening areas or islands of columnar epithelium, with no signs of cervical carcinogenesis (Figure 1.14a). It is termed an abnormal or atypical transformation zone (ATZ) when evidence of cervical carcinogenesis such as dysplastic change is observed in the transformation zone (Figure 1.14b). Identifying the transformation zone is of great importance in colposcopy, as almost all manifestations of cervical carcinogenesis occur in this zone.

Congenital transformation zone

During early embryonic life, the cuboidal epithelium of the vaginal tube is replaced by the squamous epithelium, which begins at the caudal end of the dorsal urogenital sinus. This process is completed well before birth and the entire length of vagina and the ectocervix is meant to be covered by squamous epithelium. This process proceeds very rapidly along the lateral walls, and later in the anterior and posterior vaginal walls. If the epithelialization proceeds normally, the original squamocolumnar junction will be located at the external os at birth. On the other hand, if this process is arrested for some reason or incomplete, the original squamocolumnar junction will be located distal to the external os or may rarely be located on the vaginal walls, particularly involving the anterior and posterior fornices. The cuboidal epithelium remaining here will undergo squamous metaplasia. This late conversion to squamous epithelium in the anterior and posterior vaginal walls, as well as the ectocervix, results in the formation of the congenital transformation zone. Thus, it is a variant of intrauterine squamous metaplasia, in which differentiation of the squamous epithelium is not fully completed due to an interference with normal maturation. Excessive maturation is seen on the surface (as evidenced by keratinization) with delayed, incomplete maturation in deeper layers. Clinically, it may be seen as an extensive whitish-grey, hyperkeratotic area extending from the anterior and posterior lips of the cervix to the vaginal fornices. Gradual maturation of the epithelium may occur over several years. This type of transformation zone is seen in less than 5 % of women and is a variant of the normal transformation zone.

Chapter 2

An introduction to cervical intraepithelial neoplasia (CIN)

- Invasive squamous cell cervical cancers are preceded by a long phase of preinvasive disease, collectively referred to as cervical intraepithelial neoplasia (CIN).

- CIN may be categorized into grades 1, 2 and 3 depending upon the proportion of the thickness of the epithelium showing mature and differentiated cells.

- More severe grades of CIN (2 and 3) reveal a greater proportion of the thickness of the epithelium composed of undifferentiated cells.

- Persistent infection with one or more of the oncogenic subtypes of human papillomaviruses (HPV) is a necessary cause for cervical neoplasia.

- Most cervical abnormalities caused by HPV infection are unlikely to progress to high-grade CIN or cervical cancer.

- Most low-grade CIN regress within relatively short periods or do not progress to high-grade lesions.

- High-grade CIN carries a much higher probability of progressing to invasive cancer.

- The precursor lesion arising from the columnar epithelium is referred to as adenocarcinoma *in situ* (AIS). AIS may be associated with CIN in one-to two-thirds of cases.

Invasive cervical cancers are usually preceded by a long phase of preinvasive disease. This is characterized microscopically as a spectrum of events progressing from cellular atypia to various grades of dysplasia or cervical intraepithelial neoplasia (CIN) before progression to invasive carcinoma. A good knowledge of the etiology, pathophysiology and natural history of CIN provides a strong basis both for visual testing and for colposcopic diagnosis and understanding the principles of treatment of these lesions. This chapter describes the evolution of the classification systems of cervical squamous cell cancer precursors, the cytological and histological basis of their diagnosis, as well as their natural history in terms of regression, persistence and progression rates. It also describes the precancerous lesions arising in the cervical columnar epithelium, commonly referred to as glandular lesions.

The concept of cervical cancer precursors dates back to the late nineteenth century, when areas of non-invasive atypical epithelial changes were recognized in tissue specimens adjacent to invasive cancers (William, 1888). The term carcinoma *in situ* (CIS) was introduced in 1932 to denote those lesions in which the undifferentiated carcinomatous cells involved the full thickness of the epithelium, without disruption of the basement membrane (Broders, 1932). The association between CIS and invasive cervical cancer was subsequently reported. The term dysplasia was introduced in the late 1950s to designate the cervical epithelial atypia that is intermediate between the normal epithelium and CIS (Reagan *et al.*, 1953). Dysplasia was further categorized into three groups – mild, moderate and severe – depending on the degree of involvement of the epithelial thickness by the atypical cells. Subsequently, for many years, cervical precancerous lesions were reported using the categories of dysplasia and CIS, and are still widely used in many developing countries.

A system of classification with separate classes for dysplasia and CIS was increasingly perceived as an arbitrary configuration, based upon the findings from a number of follow-up studies involving women with such lesions. It was observed that some cases of dysplasia regressed, some persisted and others progressed to CIS. A direct correlation with progression and histological grade was observed. These observations led to the concept of a single, continuous disease process by which normal epithelium evolves into epithelial precursor lesions and on to invasive cancer. On the basis of the above observations, the term cervical intraepithelial neoplasia (CIN) was introduced in 1968 to denote the whole range of cellular atypia confined to the epithelium. CIN was divided into grades 1, 2 and 3 (Richart 1968). CIN 1 corresponded to mild dysplasia, CIN 2 to moderate dysplasia, and CIN 3 corresponded to both severe dysplasia and CIS.

In the 1980s, the pathological changes such as koilocytic or condylomatous atypia associated with human papillomavirus (HPV) infection were increasingly recognized. Koilocytes are atypical cells with a perinuclear cavitation or halo in the cytoplasm indicating the cytopathic changes due to HPV infection. This led to the development of a simplified two-grade histological system. Thus, in 1990, a histopathological terminology based on two grades of disease was proposed: low-grade CIN comprising the abnormalities consistent with koilocytic atypia and CIN 1 lesions and high-grade CIN comprising CIN 2 and 3. The high-grade lesions were considered to be true precursors of invasive cancer (Richart 1990).

In 1988, the US National Cancer Institute convened a workshop to propose a new scheme for reporting cervical cytology results (NCI workshop report, 1989; Solomon, 1989; Kurman *et al.*, 1991). The recommendations from this workshop and the subsequent revision in a second workshop held in 1991 became known as the Bethesda system (TBS) (NCI workshop report, 1992). The main feature of TBS was the creation of the term squamous intraepithelial lesion (SIL), and a two-grade scheme consisting of low-grade (LSIL) and high-grade (HSIL) lesions. TBS classification combines flat condylomatous (HPV)

Table 2.1: Correlation between dysplasia/carcinoma *in situ*, cervical intraepithelial neoplasia (CIN) and the Bethesda terminology

Dysplasia terminology	Original CIN terminology	Modified CIN terminology	The Bethesda system (SIL) terminology (1991)
Normal	Normal	Normal	Within normal limits Benign cellular changes (infection or repair)
Atypia			ASCUS/AGUS
	Koilocytic atypia, flat condyloma, without epithelial changes	Low-grade CIN	LSIL
Mild dysplasia or mild dyskaryosis	CIN 1	Low-grade CIN	LSIL
Moderate dysplasia or moderate dyskaryosis	CIN 2	High-grade CIN	HSIL
Severe dysplasia or severe dyskaryosis	CIN 3	High-grade CIN	HSIL
Carcinoma *in-situ*	CIN 3	High-grade CIN	HSIL
Invasive carcinoma	Invasive carcinoma	Invasive carcinoma	Invasive carcinoma

CIN: cervical intraepithelial neoplasia; LSIL: Low-grade squamous intraepithelial lesion; HSIL: High-grade squamous intraepithelial lesion; ASCUS: Atypical squamous cells of undetermined significance; AGUS: Atypical glandular cells of undetermined significance

changes and low-grade CIN (CIN 1) into LSIL, while the HSIL encompasses more advanced CIN such as CIN 2 and 3. The term lesion was used to emphasize that any of the morphological changes upon which a diagnosis is based do not necessarily identify a neoplastic process. Though designed for cytological reporting, TBS is also used to report histopathology findings. TBS is predominantly used in North America. The correlation between the dysplasia/carcinoma *in situ* terminology and the various grades of CIN, as well as TBS, are given in Table 2.1. We use the CIN terminology in discussing the various grades of cervical squamous precancerous lesions in this manual.

TBS was reevaluated and revised in a 2001 workshop convened by the National Cancer Institute, USA, cosponsored by 44 professional societies representing more than 20 countries (Solomon *et al.*, 2002). The reporting categories under the 2001 Bethesda System are summarized in Table 2.2.

Clinical features of CIN

There are no specific symptoms and no characteristic clinical features that indicate the presence of CIN. Many of these lesions, however, may turn white on application of 3-5% acetic acid, and may be iodine-negative on application of Lugol's iodine solution, as the CIN epithelium contains little or no glycogen.

Diagnosis and grading of CIN by cytology

CIN may be identified by microscopic examination of cervical cells in a cytology smear stained by the Papanicolaou technique. In cytological preparations, individual cell changes are assessed for the diagnosis of CIN and its grading. In contrast, histological examination of whole tissues allows several other features to be examined. Cytological assessment of CIN, based on nuclear and cytoplasmic changes is often quite challenging (Figure 2.1).

Table 2.2: The 2001 Bethesda System: Reporting categories

Negative for intraepithelial lesion or malignancy
Epithelial cell abnormalities
  Squamous cell
    Atypical squamous cells (ASC)
      'of undetermined significance' (ASC-US)
      'cannot exclude HSIL' (ASC-H)
    Low-grade squamous intraepithelial lesion (LSIL)
    High-grade squamous intraepithelial lesion (HSIL)
    Squamous cell carcinoma
  Glandular
    Atypical glandular cells (AGC)
    (*specify endocervical, endometrial, or not otherwise specified*)
    Atypical glandular cells, favour neoplastic
    (*specify endocervical, or not otherwise specified*)
    Endocervical adenocarcinoma *in situ* (AIS)
    Adenocarcinoma
  Other (list not comprehensive)
    Endometrial cells in a woman over 40 years of age

Nuclear enlargement with variation in size and shape is a regular feature of all dysplastic cells (Figure 2.1). Increased intensity of staining (hyperchromasia) is another prominent feature. Irregular chromatin distribution with clumping is always present in dysplastic cells. Mitotic figures and visible nucleoli are uncommon in cytological smears. Abnormal nuclei in superficial or intermediate cells indicate a low-grade CIN, whereas abnormality in nuclei of parabasal and basal cells indicates high-grade CIN. The amount of

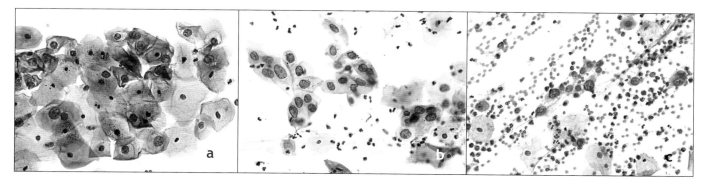

FIGURE 2.1: Cytological appearance of (a) CIN 1, (b) CIN 2, (c) CIN 3 (x20).

cytoplasm in relation to the size of the nucleus (nuclear-cytoplasmic ratio) is one of the most important base for assessing the grade of CIN (Figure 2.1). Increased ratios are associated with more severe degrees of CIN. More often than not, a cervical smear contains cells with a range of changes; considerable challenges and subjectivity, therefore, are involved in reporting the results. Experience of the cytologist is critically important in final reporting.

Diagnosis and grading of CIN by histopathology

CIN may be suspected through cytological examination using the Papanicolaou technique or through

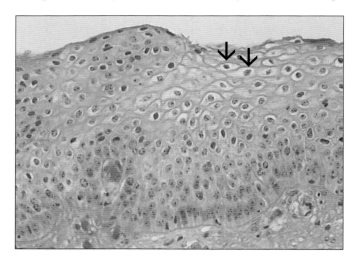

FIGURE 2.2: Histology of CIN 1: Note that the dysplastic cells are confined to the lower third of the epithelium. Koilocytes indicated by arrows are observed mostly in the upper layers of the epithelium (x20).

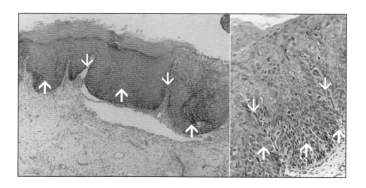

FIGURE 2.3: Histology of CIN 2: Atypical cells are found mostly in the lower two-thirds of the epithelium. Note the rete pegs indicated by the heavy arrows. Note the stretched out capillaries in the stromal papillae indicated by the narrow arrows

colposcopic examination. Final diagnosis of CIN is established by the histopathological examination of a cervical punch biopsy or excision specimen. A judgement of whether or not a cervical tissue specimen reveals CIN, and to what degree, is dependent on the histological features concerned with differentiation, maturation and stratification of cells and nuclear abnormalities. The proportion of the thickness of the epithelium showing mature and differentiated cells is used for grading CIN. More severe degrees of CIN are likely to have a greater proportion of the thickness of epithelium composed of undifferentiated cells, with only a narrow layer of mature, differentiated cells on the surface.

Nuclear abnormalities such as enlarged nuclei, increased nuclear-cytoplasmic ratio, increased intensity of nuclear staining (hyperchromasia), nuclear polymorphism and variation in nuclear size (anisokaryosis) are assessed when a diagnosis is being made. There is often a strong correlation between the proportion of epithelium revealing maturation and the degree of nuclear abnormality. Mitotic figures are seen in cells that are in cell division; they are infrequent in normal epithelium and, if present, they are seen only in the parabasal layer. As the severity of CIN increases, the number of mitotic figures also increases; these may be seen in the superficial layers of the epithelium. The less differentiation in an epithelium, the higher the level at which mitotic figures are likely to be seen. Abnormal configurations of mitotic figures also are taken into account in arriving at final diagnosis.

In CIN 1 there is good maturation with minimal nuclear abnormalities and few mitotic figures (Figure 2.2). Undifferentiated cells are confined to the deeper layers (lower third) of the epithelium. Mitotic figures are present, but not very numerous. Cytopathic changes due to HPV infection may be observed in the full thickness of the epithelium.

CIN 2 is characterized by dysplastic cellular changes mostly restricted to the lower half or the lower two-thirds of the epithelium, with more marked nuclear abnormalities than in CIN 1 (Figure 2.3). Mitotic figures may be seen throughout the lower half of the epithelium.

In CIN 3, differentiation and stratification may be totally absent or present only in the superficial quarter of the epithelium with numerous mitotic figures (Figures 2.4 and 2.5). Nuclear abnormalities extend throughout the thickness of the epithelium. Many mitotic figures have abnormal forms.

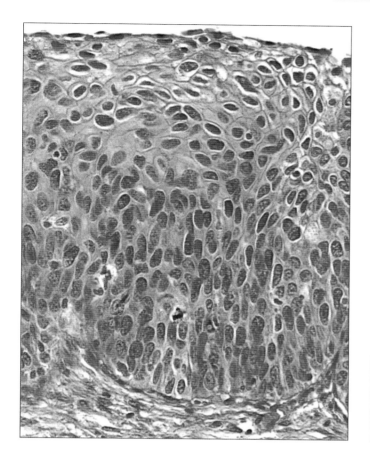

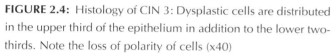

FIGURE 2.4: Histology of CIN 3: Dysplastic cells are distributed in the upper third of the epithelium in addition to the lower two-thirds. Note the loss of polarity of cells (x40)

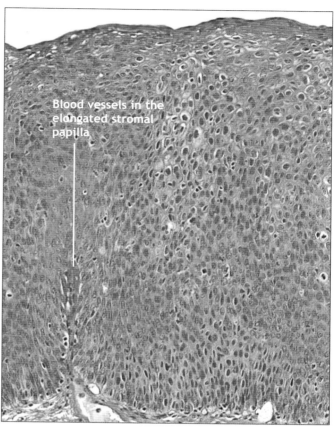

FIGURE 2.5: Histology of CIN 3: Dysplastic cells are distributed in the full thickness of the epithelium with loss of polarity of cells (x20)

A close interaction between cytologists, histopathologists and colposcopists improves reporting in all three disciplines. This particularly helps in differentiating milder degrees of CIN from other conditions with which there can be confusion.

Etiopathogenesis of cervical neoplasia

Epidemiological studies have identified a number of risk factors that contribute to the development of cervical cancer precursors and cervical cancer. These include infection with certain oncogenic types of human papillomaviruses (HPV), sexual intercourse at an early age, multiple sexual partners, multiparity, long-term oral contraceptive use, tobacco smoking, low socioeconomic status, infection with *Chlamydia trachomatis*, micronutrient deficiency and a diet deficient in vegetables and fruits (IARC, 1995; Bosch *et al.*, 1995; Schiffman *et al.*, 1996; Walboomers *et al.*, 1999; Franco *et al.*, 1999; Ferenczy & Franco, 2002).

HPV types 16, 18, 31, 33, 35, 39, 45, 51, 52, 56, 58, 59 and 68 are strongly associated with CIN and invasive cancer (IARC, 1995; Walboomers *et al.*, 1999). Persistent infection with one or more of the above oncogenic types is considered to be a necessary cause for cervical neoplasia (IARC, 1995). The pooled analysis of results from a multicentre case-control study conducted by the International Agency for Research on Cancer (IARC, 1995) revealed relative risks (RR) ranging from 17 in Colombia to 156 in the Philippines, with a pooled RR of 60 (95% confidence interval: 49-73) for cervical cancer (Walboomers *et al.*, 1999). The association was equally strong for squamous cell carcinoma (RR: 62) and adenocarcinoma of the cervix (RR: 51). HPV DNA was detected in 99.7% of 1000 evaluable cervical cancer biopsy specimens obtained from 22 countries (Walboomers *et al.*, 1999; Franco *et al.*, 1999). HPV 16 and 18 are the main viral genotypes found in cervical cancers worldwide.

Several cohort (follow-up) studies have reported a strong association between persistent oncogenic HPV infection and high risk of developing CIN (Koutsky *et al.*, 1992; Ho *et al.*, 1995; Ho *et al.*, 1998; Moscicki *et al.*, 1998; Liaw *et al.*, 1999; Wallin *et al.*, 1999;

Moscicki *et al.*, 2001; Woodman *et al.*, 2001; Schlecht *et al.*, 2002).

HPV infection is transmitted through sexual contact and the risk factors therefore are closely related to sexual behaviour (e.g., lifetime number of sexual partners, sexual intercourse at an early age). In most women, HPV infections are transient. The natural history of HPV infection has been extensively reviewed. Although the prevalence of HPV infection varies in different regions of the world, it generally reaches a peak of about 20-30% among women aged 20-24 years, with a subsequent decline to approximately 3-10% among women aged over 30 (Herrero *et al.*, 1997a; Herrero *et al.*, 1997b; Sellors *et al.*, 2000). About 80% of young women who become infected with HPV have transient infections that clear up within 12-18 months (Ho *et al.*, 1998; Franco *et al.*, 1999; Thomas *et al.*, 2000; Liaw *et al.*, 2001).

HPV infection is believed to start in the basal cells or parabasal cells of the metaplastic epithelium. If the infection persists, integration of viral genome into the host cellular genome may occur. The normal differentiation and maturation of the immature squamous metaplastic into the mature squamous metaplastic epithelium may be disrupted as a result of expression of E6/E7 oncoproteins and the loss of normal growth control. This may then lead to development of abnormal dysplastic epithelium. If the neoplastic process continues uninterrupted, the early low-grade lesions may eventually involve the full thickness of the epithelium. Subsequently the disease may traverse the basement membrane and become invasive cancer, extending to surrounding tissues and organs. The invasion may then affect blood and lymphatic vessels and the disease may spread to the lymph nodes and distant organs.

Natural history of cervical cancer precursors

Despite women's frequent exposure to HPV, development of cervical neoplasia is uncommon. Most cervical abnormalities caused by HPV infection are unlikely to progress to high-grade CIN or cervical cancer, as most of them regress by themselves. The long time frame between initial infection and overt disease indicates that several cofactors (e.g., genetic differences, hormonal effects, micronutrient deficiencies, smoking, or chronic inflammation) may be necessary for disease progression. Spontaneous regression of CIN may also indicate that many women may not be exposed to these cofactors.

Several studies have addressed the natural history of CIN, with particular emphasis on disease regression, persistence and progression (McIndoe *et al.*, 1984; Östor *et al.*, 1993; Mitchell *et al.*, 1994; Melinkow *et al.*, 1998; Holowaty *et al.*, 1999). They have revealed that most low-grade lesions are transient; most of them regress to normal within relatively short periods or do not progress to more severe forms. High-grade CIN, on the other hand, carries a much higher probability of progressing to invasive cancer, although a proportion of such lesions also regress or persist. It is appears that the mean interval for progression of cervical precursors to invasive cancer is some 10 to 20 years.

A few studies have attempted to summarize the rates of regression, persistence and progression of CIN. Even though these studies have many limitations, they provide interesting insight into the biological behaviour of these lesions. The results of a pooled analysis of studies published from 1950 to 1993 are given in Table 2.3 (Östor *et al.*, 1993). In another overview, the cumulative probabilities for all grades of CIN that had been followed by both cytology and histology were 45% for regression, 31% for persistence, and 23% for progression (Mitchell *et al.*, 1994). Progression rates to invasive cancer for studies following up CIS patients by biopsy ranged from 29 to 36% (McIndoe *et al.*, 1984). A meta analysis of 27 000 women gave the weighted average rates of progression to HSIL and invasive cancer at 24 months according to baseline cytological abnormality given in Table 2.4 (Melinkow *et al.*, 1998).

Table 2.3: Regression, persistence and progression probabilities of CIN

CIN category	Regression	Persistence	Progression to CIN 3	Progression to invasive cancer
CIN 1	57%	32%	11%	1%
CIN 2	43%	35%	22%	1.5%
CIN 3	32%	56%	-	12%

Table 2.4: Natural history of SIL

Baseline cytological abnormality	Regression to normal at 24 months	Progression to HSIL at 24 months	Progression to invasive cancer at 24 months
ASCUS	68.2%	7.1%	0.3%
LSIL	47.4%	20.8%	0.2%
HSIL	35.0%	23.4% (persistence)	1.4%

Holowaty *et al.*, (1999) calculated RR of progression and regression by 2-years of follow-up for moderate and severe dysplasias, with mild dysplasia taken as the baseline reference category. RRs for CIS were 8.1 for moderate dysplasia and 22.7 for severe dysplasia. The corresponding RRs for invasive cancer were 4.5 and 20.7, respectively.

Adenocarcinoma *in situ*

The precursor lesion that has been recognized to arise from the columnar epithelium is referred to as adenocarcinoma *in situ* (AIS). In AIS, normal columnar epithelium is replaced by abnormal epithelium showing loss of polarity, increased cell size, increased nuclear size, nuclear hyperchromasia, mitotic activity, reduction of cytoplasmic mucin expression and cellular stratification or piling (Figure 2.6). Abnormal branching and budding glands with intraluminal papillary epithelial projections lacking stromal cores may also be observed. It may be sub-divided based on the cell types into endocervical, endometroid,

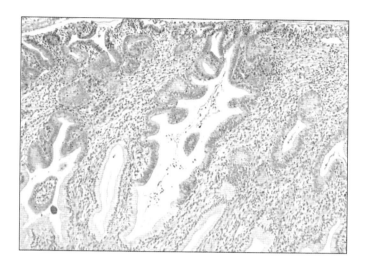

FIGURE 2.6: Adenocarcinoma *in situ,* coexisting with a normal endocervical epithelium (x10).

intestinal and mixed cell types. The majority of AIS are found in the transformation zone. AIS may be associated with CIN of the squamous epithelium in one- to two-thirds of cases.

Chapter 3

An introduction to invasive cancer of the uterine cervix

- Preclinical invasive cancer refers to early cervical cancer, with minimal stromal invasion, often without any symptoms or clinical features.

- As the stromal invasion progresses, the disease becomes clinically obvious, revealing several growth patterns visible on speculum examination.

- Histologically 90-95% of invasive cervical cancers are squamous cell cancers; adenocarcinoma constitutes less than 5% of cervical cancers in most developing countries.

- The most widely used staging system for invasive cervical cancer is based on tumour size and the spread of disease into the vagina, parametrium, urinary bladder, rectum and distant organs.

- Clinical stage of disease at presentation is the single most important predictor of survival from invasive cervical cancer.

This chapter deals with the clinical features and diagnosis of invasive cervical carcinoma. The diagnosis of invasive cervical cancer may be suggested by abnormal physical findings on speculum and vaginal examination and may be confirmed by histological examination of tissue specimens. In a proportion of these cancers no symptoms and gross abnormal findings are seen on physical examination and these are called preclinical invasive cervical cancers. Colposcopy has an important role to play in the diagnosis of preclinical early invasive cancer.

Clinical features

Women with invasive cervical cancer often present with one or more of the following symptoms: intermenstrual bleeding, postcoital bleeding, heavier menstrual flows, excessive seropurulent discharge, foul smelling discharge, recurrent cystitis, urinary frequency and urgency, backache, and lower abdominal pain. In advanced stages, patients may present with breathlessness due to severe anaemia, obstructive uropathy, oedema of the lower limbs, haematuria, bowel obstruction and cachexia. Vaginal speculum examination reveals an ulceroproliferative growth in most women.

In very early phases of stromal invasion, cervical cancer may not generate any obvious symptoms or clinical features, and, therefore, is known as preclinical invasive disease. The earliest form of invasive cancer is histologically recognized as microinvasive carcinoma: cancers that have invaded no more than 5 mm deep and 7 mm wide into the underlying cervical stroma. Early invasive cancers appear as a tiny bud of invasive cells that have penetrated through the basement membrane and pushed into the underlying stroma (Figures 3.1 and 3.2). Evidence of stromal reaction to invasion in the form of localized lymphocytic collection or loosening of the stroma surrounding the invasion may also be evident.

As the stromal invasion progresses, the disease becomes clinically obvious, with several growth patterns, which are often visible on speculum examination. Very early lesions may present as a rough, reddish, granular area that bleeds on touch (Figure 3.3). More advanced cancers can be exophytic, endophytic or a combination of both (Figures 3.4-3.6). Exophytic carcinomas are usually superficially invasive and their bulk grows into the vaginal lumen as a

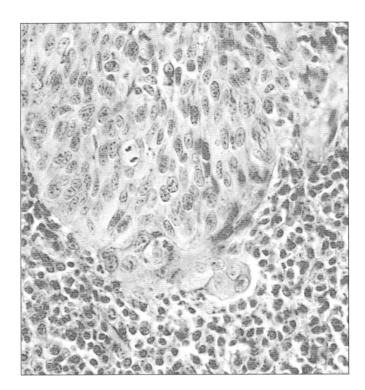

FIGURE 3.1: Histology – early stromal invasion (x 40)

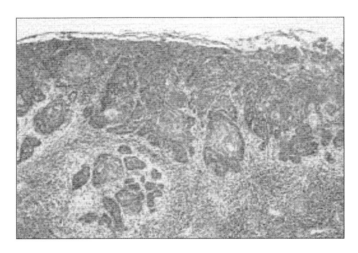

FIGURE 3.2: Histology – early stromal invasion (x 10)

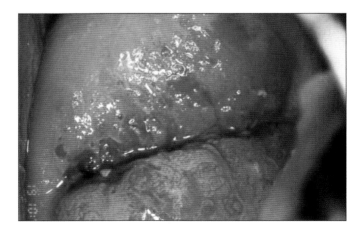

FIGURE 3.3: Early invasive cervical cancer

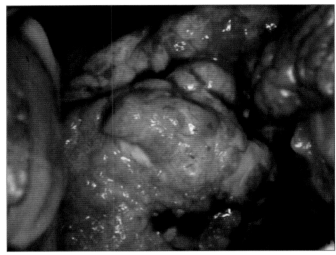

FIGURE 3.4: Invasive cervical cancer

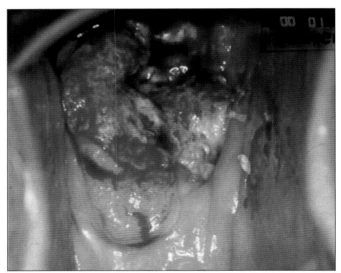

FIGURE 3.5: Invasive cervical cancer

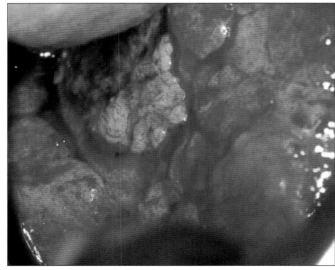

FIGURE 3.6: Advanced invasive cervical cancer with ulceroproliferative growth

mushroom or proliferating, bulging cauliflower-like growth with polypoid or papillary excrescences. Endophytic cancers may extensively infiltrate the stroma, distorting the cervix, without much visible surface growth. These lesions may expand into the endocervix leaving the squamous epithelium of the cervix intact until the lesions exceed 5-6 cm in a diameter. They result in a grossly enlarged, irregular barrel-shaped cervix with a rough, papillary or granular surface. Such cancers may remain silent for a long time. Partly exophytic and endophytic tumours are usually ulcerated with deep infiltration of the underlying stroma. In all types, bleeding on touch and necrosis are predominant clinical features. Foul-smelling discharge is also common due to superadded anaerobic infection of the necrotic tissue.

As the invasion continues further, it may directly involve the vagina, parametrium, pelvic sidewall, bladder and rectum. Compression of the ureter due to advanced local disease causes ureteral obstruction with resulting hydronephrosis (enlargement of kidneys) and, ultimately, renal failure. Regional lymph node metastasis occurs along with local invasion. Metastatic cancer in para-aortic nodes may extend through the node capsule and directly invade the vertebrae and nerve roots. Direct invasion of the branches of the sciatic nerve roots causes back pain, and encroachment of the pelvic wall veins and lymphatics causes oedema of the lower limbs. Haematogenous spread to lumbar vertebrae and psoas muscle may occur without nodal disease. Distant metastases occur late in the disease, usually involving para-aortic nodes, lungs, liver, bone and other structures.

Microscopic pathology

Histologically, approximately 90-95% of invasive cervical cancers arising from the uterine cervix in developing countries are squamous cell cancers (Figures 3.7 and 3.8) and 2 to 8% are adenocarcinomas (Figure 3.9).

Microscopically, most squamous cell carcinomas appear as infiltrating networks of bands of neoplastic cells with intervening stroma, with a great deal of variation in growth pattern, cell type and degree of differentiation. The cervical stroma separating the bands of malignant cells is infiltrated by lymphocytes and plasma cells. These malignant cells may be subdivided into keratinizing and non-keratinizing types. The tumours may be well, moderately or poorly differentiated carcinomas. Approximately 50-60% are moderately differentiated cancers and the remainder are evenly distributed between the well and poorly differentiated categories.

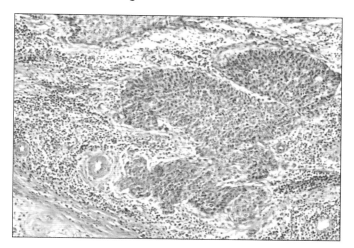

FIGURE 3.8: Histology – Non-keratinizing invasive squamous cell carcinoma (x 10)

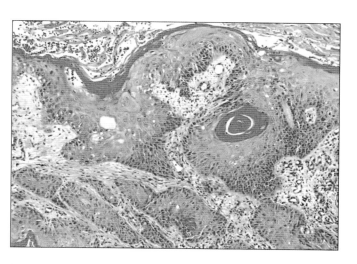

FIGURE 3.7: Histology – Keratinizing well differentiated invasive squamous cell carcinoma (x 10)

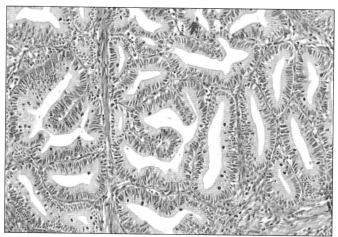

FIGURE 3.9: Histology – Well differentiated invasive adenocarcinoma (x 20)

23

Keratinizing squamous cell carcinoma is composed of characteristic whorls of epidermoid cells containing central nests of keratin (keratin pearls) (Figure 3.7). The nuclei are large and hyperchromatic with coarse chromatin. Intercellular bridges are visible, along with keratohyaline granules and cytoplasmic keratinization. Only few mitotic figures are visible.

Non-keratinizing squamous cell carcinoma (Figure 3.8) appears as irregular, jagged nests of plump polygonal cells invading the cervical stroma. There may be dyskeratosis and intercellular bridges. Cellular and nuclear polymorphism is more obvious and mitotic figures are quite numerous. Keratin pearls are usually absent.

Other uncommon types of squamous cell carcinoma include condylomatous squamous cell carcinoma (also called verrucous carcinoma), papillary squamous cell carcinoma, lymphoepithelioma-like carcinoma, and squamotransitional cell carcinoma.

In many developing countries, adenocarcinoma constitutes less than 5% of all cervical cancers. More often than not, it arises in the endocervical canal from the glandular epithelium. The most common form of adenocarcinoma is the endocervical cell type, where the abnormal glands are of various shapes and sizes with budding and branching (Figure 3.9). Most of these tumours are well to moderately differentiated. The glandular elements are arranged in a complex pattern. Papillae may project into the gland lumen and from the surface. Some of the cells may contain a moderate to large amount of mucin.

The other types of adenocarcinoma include intestinal-type, signet-ring cell adenocarcinoma, adenoma malignum, villoglandular papillary adenocarcinoma, endometroid adenocarcinoma and papillary serous adenocarcinoma. Adenosquamous carcinoma includes tumours with glandular and squamous growth patterns.

The presence of tumour cells within the lumen of a capillary space is evidence of aggressive growth potential in both squamous cell and adenocarcinoma of the cervix, and has been correlated with increased risk for regional lymph node metastasis. Invasion of blood vessels occasionally occurs and is a particularly poor prognostic sign, correlating with distant, blood-borne metastasis. Though the cytological features associated with invasive squamous cell carcinoma of the cervix have been well described, cytology is not a reliable method of diagnosing invasive lesions. Identifying these lesions in cytology smears requires extensive experience, as the cervical smear often contains only very few malignant cells among an assortment of debris and red blood cells. Adenocarcinoma of the cervix is often not recognized by cytologists; an experienced cytologist is able to recognize it when the cellular features are at extreme variance compared to normal. The recognition of individual cell types is even more complex. Hence, the final confirmatory diagnosis of an invasive cancer is always based on histopathology. A tissue specimen taken from the periphery of the growth is preferred for diagnosis, as this is more likely to contain morphologically intact tumour tissue, whereas a biopsy specimen taken from the centre of a growth may contain necrotic material which will compromise the accuracy of histological diagnosis.

Staging

Treatment planning and assessment of prognosis requires detailed evaluation of the patient's general health and the determination of the clinical stage of invasive cancer. The widely used staging system for cervical cancer was developed by the International Federation of Gynecology and Obstetrics (FIGO), and is given in Table 3.1. This is primarily a clinical staging system based on tumour size and extension of the disease in the pelvis. The extent of growth of cancer is assessed clinically, as well as by various investigations to categorize the disease stages I through IV (Table 3.1 and Figure 3.10). Stage I represents growth localized to the cervix, while stage IV represents the growth phase in which the cancer has spread to distant organs by metastases.

The FIGO staging is assessed using methods including inspection and palpation by vaginal and rectal examination, colposcopy, cystoscopy, endocervical curettage, hysteroscopy, intravenous urogram, and chest and skeletal X-rays. Lymphangiography, ultrasonography, computerized tomography (CT) and magnetic resonance imaging (MRI) and laparoscopy may provide additional information, but this information should not be used to assess the FIGO clinical stages, despite the fact that these investigations may provide valuable information for planning treatment. In many low-resource settings, however, speculum examination, per vaginal and per rectal examination are the only feasible approaches to staging. Cystoscopy and radiological assessment with chest and skeletal X-rays and intravenous urograms may additionally be carried out if possible. Staging should routinely be carried out

Table 3.1: FIGO staging (See Figure 3.10)

Stage I

Stage I is carcinoma strictly confined to the cervix; extension to the uterine corpus should be disregarded. The diagnosis of both Stages IA1 and IA2 should be based on microscopic examination of removed tissue, preferably a cone, which must include the entire lesion.

Stage IA: Invasive cancer identified only microscopically. Invasion is limited to measured stromal invasion with a maximum depth of 5 mm and no wider than 7 mm.

Stage IA1:   Measured invasion of the stroma no greater than 3 mm in depth and no wider than 7 mm diameter.

Stage IA2:   Measured invasion of stroma greater than 3 mm but no greater than 5 mm in depth and no wider than 7 mm in diameter.

Stage IB: Clinical lesions confined to the cervix or preclinical lesions greater than Stage IA. All gross lesions even with superficial invasion are Stage IB cancers.

Stage IB1:   Clinical lesions no greater than 4 cm in size.

Stage IB2:   Clinical lesions greater than 4 cm in size.

Stage II

Stage II is carcinoma that extends beyond the cervix, but does not extend to the pelvic wall. The carcinoma involves the vagina, but not as far as the lower third.

Stage IIA: No obvious parametrial involvement. Involvement of up to the upper two-thirds of the vagina.

Stage IIB: Obvious parametrial involvement, but not to the pelvic sidewall.

Stage III

Stage III is carcinoma that has extended to the pelvic sidewall. On rectal examination, there is no cancer-free space between the tumour and the pelvic sidewall. The tumour involves the lower third of the vagina. All cases with hydronephrosis or a non-functioning kidney are Stage III cancers.

Stage IIIA: No extension to the pelvic sidewall but involvement of the lower third of the vagina.

Stage IIIB: Extension to the pelvic sidewall or hydronephrosis or non-functioning kidney.

Stage IV

Stage IV is carcinoma that has extended beyond the true pelvis or has clinically involved the mucosa of the bladder and/or rectum.

Stage IVA: Spread of the tumour into adjacent pelvic organs.

Stage IVB: Spread to distant organs.

It is impossible to estimate clinically whether a cancer of the cervix has extended to the corpus. The determination of the extension to the corpus should therefore be disregarded.

and documented in the case record with a descriptive diagram whenever an invasive cervical cancer is discovered. The investigations and procedures, on the basis of which the staging assessment was carried out, should also be described.

Treatment and prognosis

The standard treatment of cervical cancer may involve surgery or radiotherapy or a combination of both. Early cervical cancers (stage I and IIA) may be treated by either procedure. Radiotherapy is the treatment of

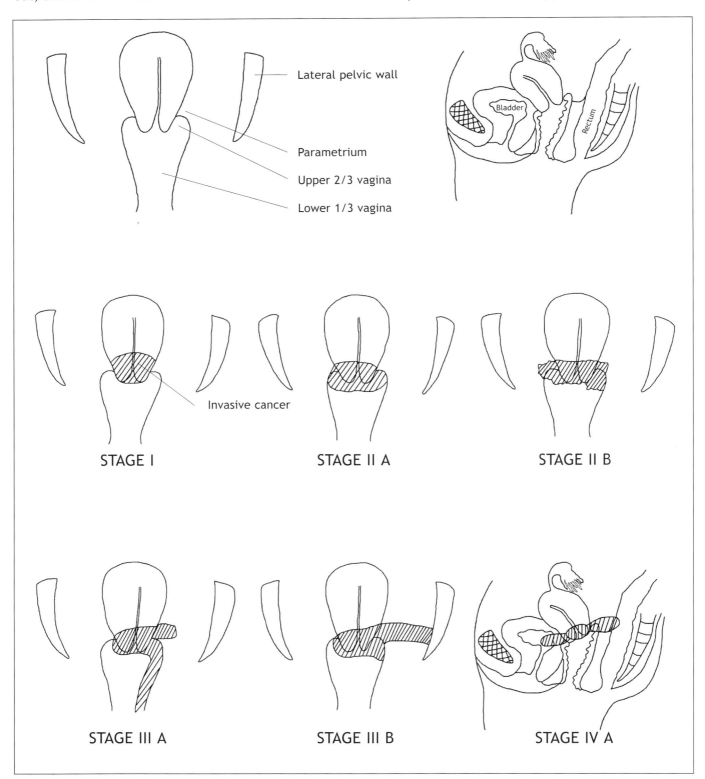

FIGURE 3.10: A schematic diagram of clinical stages of invasive cancer of the cervix

choice once the disease has spread beyond the confines of the cervix and vaginal fornices, when surgery is not effective. The management of cervical cancer with radiotherapy may often involve a combination of external radiotherapy (for the entire pelvis) and intracavitary irradiation (to the central part of the disease). The addition of intracavitory irradiation to external beam radiotherapy is associated with improved disease control and survival, as compared to external radiotherapy alone for locally advanced disease such as stage IIB and III.

Women with microinvasive cancer (stage IA) may be treated with conization or total hysterectomy or extended hysterectomy. Those with stage IB and IIA cancer may be treated with radical (Wertheim's) hysterectomy, and pelvic lymphadenectomy or with intracavitary radiotherapy, or with a combination of external radiotherapy and intracavitary radiotherapy. In selected cases of small (< 2 cm) stage IB carcinoma, radical trachelectomy combined with laparoscopic lymphadenectomy, to salvage the reproductive function of the patient, can be performed. Radiotherapy and surgery produce similar results for early invasive cancer (stages IB and IIA). Stage IIB and III cancers are treated with a combination of external and intracavitary radiotherapy. Women with stage IV disease are treated palliatively with external radiotherapy and/or with chemotherapy.

Concomitant chemotherapy with cisplatin has improved the results of radiotherapy in advanced cervical cancer. Randomized clinical trials have shown a significant gain in overall and disease free survival for cisplatin-based therapy given concurrently with radiotherapy (Thomas, 2000; Green et al., 2001). A significant benefit of chemo-radiation on both local and distant recurrence has been observed. The absolute benefit with combined therapy in overall survival was 16%. Based on this evidence, concurrent chemotherapy with radiotherapy is emerging as the new standard of care for advanced cervical cancer.

Clinical stage of disease at presentation is the single most important predictor of long-term survival; survival rates also decline with advancing age. Other factors influencing survival include general health and nutritional status. Anaemic patients respond poorly to treatment; as do those with HIV-seropositive disease. Several clinical and population-based studies have demonstrated consistently high five-year survival associated with stage I disease (> 75%), with rapidly decreasing survival with advanced stages of disease (< 10% in stage IV) (Delgado et al., 1990; Fagundes et al., 1992; Kosary et al., 1994; Gatta et al., 1998; Sankaranarayanan et al., 1998; Denton et al., 2000). In a large series of cervical cancer patients treated by radiation therapy, the frequency of distant metastases (most frequently to para-aortic lymph nodes, lung, abdominal cavity, liver and gastrointestinal tract) was shown to increase with increasing stage of disease from 3% in stage IA to 75% in stage IVA (Fagundes et al., 1992). In a study of 1028 patients treated with radical surgery, survival rates correlated consistently with tumour volume (Burghardt et al., 1992). Five-year survival rates ranged between 91% for patients with tumours of < 2.5 cm^3 and 70% for those with tumours of 10-50 cm^3. The three-year disease-free survival ranged from 94.6% for stage I tumours $\leq$ 5 mm to 59.5% for stage I tumours $\geq$ 21 mm (Delgado et al., 1990). Advanced clinical stages are associated with increasing frequency of vascular invasion and spread to pelvic and para-aortic lymph nodes and distant metastases.

Chapter 4

An introduction to colposcopy: indications for colposcopy, instrumentation, principles, and documentation of results

- A colposcope is a low-power, stereoscopic, binocular field microscope with a powerful light source used for magnified visual examination of the uterine cervix to help in the diagnosis of cervical neoplasia.

- The most common indication of referral for colposcopy is positive screening tests (e.g., positive cytology, positive on visual inspection with acetic acid (VIA) etc.).

- The key ingredients of colposcopic examination are the observation of features of the cervical epithelium after application of normal saline, 3-5% dilute acetic acid, and Lugol's iodine solution in successive steps.

- The characteristics of acetowhite changes, if any, on the cervix following the application of dilute acetic acid are useful in colposcopic interpretation and in directing biopsies.

- The colour changes in the cervix, following the application of Lugol's iodine solution, depends on the presence or absence of glycogen in the epithelial cells. Areas containing glycogen turn brown or black; areas lacking glycogen remain colourless or pale or turn mustard or saffron yellow.

- It is important to carefully document the findings of colposcopic examination, immediately after the procedure, in a colposcopic record.

This chapter describes the indications for carrying out colposcopic examination of women, the instrumentation used for colposcopy, the basis of different colposcopic investigations and the methods of documentation of colposcopic findings. The step-by-step procedure of doing the colposcopic examination is described in the next chapter.

Indications for colposcopy

Given the availability of a colposcope and a trained colposcopist, there are a number of indications for this examination, of which positive cervical screening tests constitute the most frequent indication for colposcopy. The most common reason for referral of women for colposcopy is abnormal cervical cytology, usually discovered as a result of cytological screening (Table 4.1). Cytologically reported high-grade abnormalities such as high-grade cervical intraepithelial neoplasia

(CIN 2 and CIN 3) may be associated with an underlying invasive squamous cell cervical cancer or adenocarcinoma. It is important that all women with high-grade abnormalities be referred immediately for diagnostic colposcopy. However, there is considerable variation in the management of women with low-grade abnormalities such as low-grade cervical intraepithelial neoplasia (CIN 1).

The referral criteria in some centres, for example in developing countries where colposcopy is available, allow for the immediate referral of women with low-grade abnormalities, whereas in other regions, for example in developed countries, they are called back for repeat cytology smears every six months for up to two years and only those with persistent or progressive abnormalities are referred. It should be emphasized that women with low-grade lesions (CIN 1) on their cytology smears have a higher probability of having a

Table 4.1: Indications for colposcopy

Suspicious-looking cervix

Invasive carcinoma on cytology

CIN 2 or CIN 3 on cytology

Persisting (for more than 12-18 months) low-grade (CIN 1) abnormalities on cytology

CIN 1 on cytology

Persistently unsatisfactory quality on cytology

Infection with oncogenic human papillomaviruses (HPV)

Acetopositivity on visual inspection with acetic acid (VIA)

Acetopositivity on visual inspection with acetic acid using magnification (VIAM)

Positive on visual inspection with Lugol's iodine (VILI)

high-grade lesion that would be found at colposcopy; perhaps 15% for those with atypia and 20% with CIN 1 on cytology may harbour higher-grade lesions (Shafi *et al.*, 1997). It is advisable that women with any grade of CIN on cytology be referred for colposcopy in developing countries, in view of the possibility of reporting misclassification associated with cytology and poor compliance with follow-up.

Abnormal cytology results are tend to be quite worrying for a woman, as is a visit for a colposcopic examination. A few clinical caveats are worth mentioning. If the clinician observes characteristics of a cervix that looks suspicious, no matter what the cytology shows, it is advisable to refer the woman for colposcopic examination. Likewise, observation of an area of leukoplakia (hyperkeratosis) on the cervix should prompt a colposcopic examination, since the leukoplakia can not only obscure a lesion, but also preclude adequate cytological sampling of the area. It is still uncertain whether women with external anogenital warts are at increased risk of CIN; although it is clear that they should have routine cytology smears, it is not certain whether they would benefit from colposcopic examination (Howard *et al.*, 2001).

The potential roles of 3-5% acetic acid application and subsequent visual inspection of the cervix with magnification (VIAM) or without (VIA) and of visual

inspection with Lugol's iodine (VILI) are still under study as screening techniques (University of Zimbabwe, JHPIEGO study, 1998; Denny *et al.*, 2000; Belinson *et al.*, 2001; Sankaranarayanan *et al.*, 2001). Women who are positive for these tests may be referred for colposcopy to rule out underlying high-grade CIN and invasive cancer.

Instrumentation

Hinselmann (1925) first described the basic colposcopic equipment and its use, establishing the foundation for the practice of colposcopy. A colposcope is a low-power, stereoscopic, binocular, field microscope with a powerful variable-intensity light source that illuminates the area being examined (Figure 4.1).

The head of the colposcope, also called the 'optics carrier', contains the objective lens (at the end of the head positioned nearest to the woman being examined), two ocular lenses or eyepieces (used by the colposcopist to view the cervix), a light source, green and/or blue filters to be interposed between the light source and the objective lens, a knob to introduce the filter, a knob to change the magnification of the objective lens, if the colposcope has multiple magnification facility and a fine focusing handle. The filter is used to remove red light, to facilitate the visualization of blood vessels by making them appear

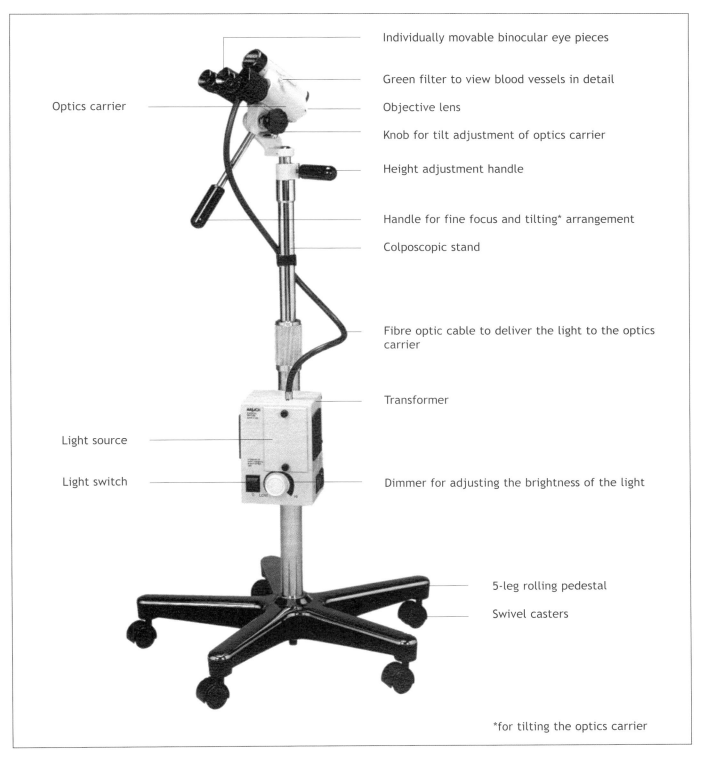

Individually movable binocular eye pieces

Green filter to view blood vessels in detail

Optics carrier

Objective lens

Knob for tilt adjustment of optics carrier

Height adjustment handle

Handle for fine focus and tilting* arrangement

Colposcopic stand

Fibre optic cable to deliver the light to the optics carrier

Transformer

Light source

Light switch

Dimmer for adjusting the brightness of the light

5-leg rolling pedestal

Swivel casters

*for tilting the optics carrier

FIGURE 4.1: Colposcope

dark. Using a knob, the head of the colposcope can be tilted up and down to facilitate examination of the cervix. The distance between the two ocular lenses can be adjusted to suit the interpupillary distance of the provider, to achieve stereoscopic vision. Each ocular lens has dioptre scales engraved on it to facilitate visual correction of individual colposcopists. The height of the head from the floor can be adjusted by using the height adjustment knob, so that colposcopy can be carried out with the colposcopist comfortably seated, without strain to the back.

Modern colposcopes usually permit adjustable magnification, commonly 6x to 40x usually in steps such as, for example, 9x, 15x, 22x. Some sophisticated

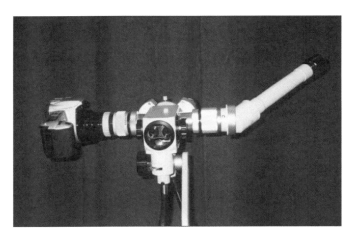

FIGURE 4.2: Colposcope with a photographic camera and a teaching side tube

and expensive equipment may have electrical zoom capability to alter the magnification. Most simple colposcopes have a single fixed magnification level such as 6x, 9x, 10x, 12x or 15x. Most of the work with a colposcope can be accomplished within the magnification range of 6x to 15x. Lower magnification yields a wider view and greater depth of field for examination of the cervix. More magnification is not necessarily better, since there are certain trade-offs as magnification increases: the field of view becomes smaller, the depth of focus dimishes, and the illumination requirement increases. However, higher magnifications may reveal finer features such as abnormal blood vessels.

The location of the light bulb in the colposcope should be easily accessible to facilitate changing them when necessary. Some colposcopes have bulbs mounted in the head of the instrument; in others, these are mounted elsewhere and the light is delivered via a fibre-optic cable to the head of the colposcope. The latter arrangement can use brighter bulbs, but less overall illumination may result if the cables are bent or twisted. A colposcope may be fitted with halogen, xenon, tungsten or incandescent bulbs. Halogen bulbs are usually preferred, as they produce strong white light. The intensity of the light source may be adjusted with a knob.

Focusing the colposcope is accomplished by adjusting the distance between the objective lens and the woman by positioning the instrument at the right working distance. Colposcopes usually have fine focus adjustments so that, if the distance between the base of the scope and the woman is kept fixed, the focus of the scope may be altered slightly using the fine focusing handle. The working distance (focal length)

between the objective lens and the patient is quite important - if it is too long (greater than 300 mm) it is hard for the colposcopist's arms to reach the woman, and if it is too short (less than 200 mm), it may be difficult to use instruments like biopsy forceps while visualizing the target with the scope. A focal distance of 250 to 300 mm is usually adequate. Changing the power of the objective lenses alters the magnification and working distance.

Colposcopes are quite heavy and are either mounted on floor pedestals with wheels, suspended from a fixed ceiling mount, or fixed to the examination table or to a wall, sometimes with a floating arm to allow for easier adjustment of position. In developing countries, it is preferable to use colposcopes mounted vertically on a floor pedestal with wheels, as they are easier to handle and can be moved within or between clinics.

Accessories such as a monocular teaching side tube, photographic camera (Figure 4.2) and CCD video camera may be added to some colposcopes. However, these substantially increase the cost of the equipment. These accessories are added using a beam splitter in most colposcopes. The beam splitter splits the light beam in half and sends the same image to the viewing port and to the accessory port. Colpophotographic systems are useful for documentation of colposcopic findings and quality control. Teaching side tubes and videocolposcopy may be useful for real-time teaching and discussion of findings. With a modern CCD camera attached to a digitalizing port, it is possible to create high-resolution digital images of the colposcopic images.

Examination table

The examination table allows the woman to be placed in a modified lithotomy position. The woman's feet may be placed either in heel rests or the legs may be supported in knee crutches. Tables or chairs that can be moved up or down mechanically or electrically are more expensive and are not absolutely necessary either for colposcopic examination or to carry out treatment procedures guided by colposcopy.

Colposcopic instruments

The instruments needed for colposcopy are few and should be placed on an instrument trolley or tray (Figure 4.3) beside the examination table. The instruments required are: bivalve specula (Figure 4.4), vaginal side-wall retractor (Figure 4.5), cotton swabs, sponge-holding forceps, long (at least 20cm long)

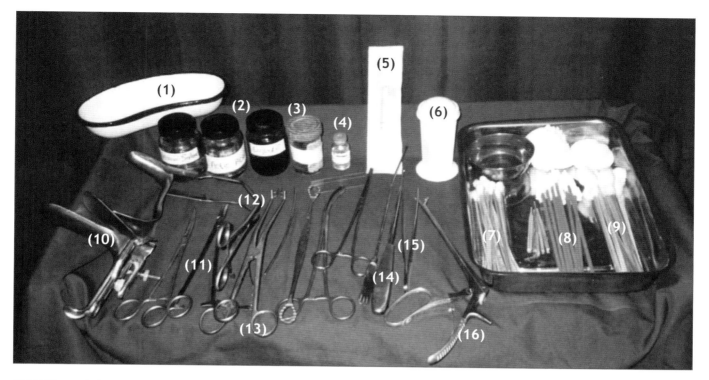

FIGURE 4.3: Colposcopy instrument tray

1: Kidney tray

2: Bottles with normal saline, 5% acetic acid and Lugol's iodine

3: Monsel's solution

4: Bottle containing formaline

5: Local anaesthetic syringe

6: Jar containing alcohol for cervical smear fixation

7: Cotton-tipped fine swab sticks

8: Cervical cytology brushes

9: Larger cotton-tipped swab sticks

10: Vaginal speculum

11: Sponge-holding forceps

12: Vaginal side-wall retractor

13: Endocervical speculum

14: Endocervical curette

15: Dissecting forceps

16: Punch biopsy forceps

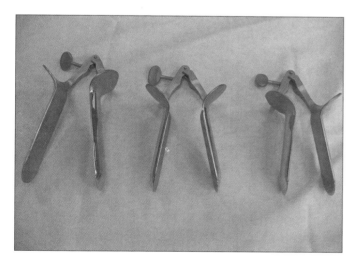

FIGURE 4.4: Collins bivalve specula of different sizes

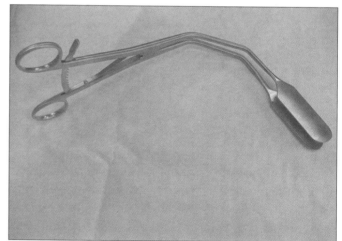

FIGURE 4.5: Vaginal side-wall retractor

anatomical dissection forceps, endocervical speculum (Figure 4.6), endocervical curette (Figure 4.7), biopsy forceps (Figure 4.8), cervical polyp forceps and single-toothed tenaculum. In addition, the instrument tray may contain instruments necessary for treatment of CIN with cryotherapy or loop electrosurgical excision procedure (LEEP) (see chapters 11 and 12). The tray should also contain the consumables used for colposcopy and treatment.

In view of the different sizes of vagina, varying widths of bivalve specula should be available. One may use Cusco's, Grave's, Collin's or Pedersen's specula.

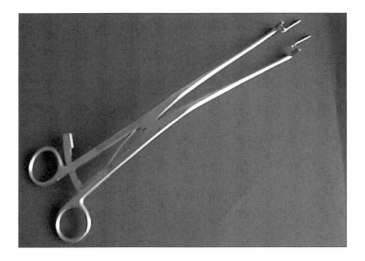

FIGURE 4.6: Endocervical speculum

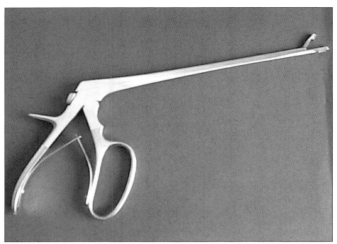

FIGURE 4.8: Cervical punch biopsy forceps with sharp, cutting edges

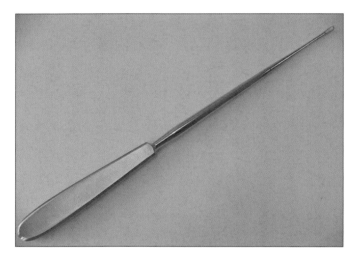

FIGURE 4.7: Endocervical curette

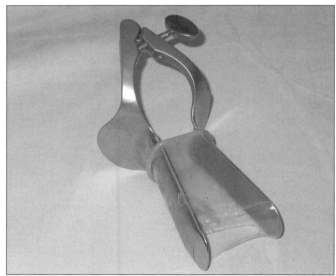

FIGURE 4.9: Vaginal speculum covered with a latex condom

One should use the widest possible speculum that can comfortably be inserted into the vagina to have optimal visualization of the cervix. Vaginal side-wall retractors are useful to prevent the lateral walls of a lax vagina from obstructing the view of the cervix. However, they may cause discomfort to the patient. An alternative approach is to use a latex condom on the speculum, the tip of which is opened with scissors 1 cm from the "nipple" (Figure 4.9). Sponge-holding forceps or long dissection forceps may be used to hold dry or moist cotton balls. The endocervical speculum or the long dissection forceps may be used to inspect the endocervical canal. The endocervical curette is used to obtain tissue specimens from the endocervix. Several

types of sharp cervical biopsy punch forceps with long shafts (20-25 cm) such as Tischler-Morgan, Townsend or Kevrokian, are available. A single-toothed tenaculum or skin (iris) hook may be used to fix the cervix when obtaining a punch biopsy. Cervical polyps may be avulsed using the polyp forceps.

Principles of colposcopy examination procedures

Saline technique

The key ingredients of colposcopic practice are the examination of the features of the cervical epithelium after application of saline, 3-5% dilute acetic acid and Lugol's iodine solution in successive steps. The study of the vascular pattern of the cervix may prove difficult after application of acetic acid and iodine solutions. Hence the application of physiological saline before acetic acid and iodine application is useful in studying the subepithelial vascular architecture in great detail. It is advisable to use a green filter to see the vessels more clearly.

Principles of acetic acid test

The other key ingredient in colposcopic practice, 3-5% acetic acid, is usually applied with a cotton applicator (cotton balls held by sponge forceps, or large rectal or small swabs) or with a small sprayer. It helps in coagulating and clearing the mucus. Acetic acid is thought to cause swelling of the epithelial tissue, columnar and any abnormal squamous epithelial areas in particular. It causes a reversible coagulation or precipitation of the nuclear proteins and cytokeratins. Thus, the effect of acetic acid depends upon the amount of nuclear proteins and cytokeratins present in the epithelium. When acetic acid is applied to normal squamous epithelium, little coagulation occurs in the superficial cell layer, as this is sparsely nucleated. Though the deeper cells contain more nuclear protein, the acetic acid may not penetrate sufficiently and, hence, the resulting precipitation is not sufficient to obliterate the colour of the underlying stroma. Areas of CIN undergo maximal coagulation due to their higher content of nuclear protein and prevent light from passing through the epithelium. As a result, the subepithelial vessel pattern is obliterated and less easy to see and the epithelium appears white. This reaction is termed acetowhitening, and produces a noticeable effect compared with the normal pinkish colour of the surrounding normal squamous epithelium of the cervix, an effect that is commonly visible to the naked eye.

With low-grade CIN, the acetic acid must penetrate into the lower one-third of the epithelium (where most of the abnormal cells with high nuclear density are located). Hence, the appearance of the whiteness is delayed and less intense due to the smaller amount of nuclear protein compared to areas with high-grade CIN or preclinical invasive cancer. Areas of high-grade CIN and invasive cancer turn densely white and opaque immediately after application of acetic acid, due to their higher concentration of abnormal nuclear protein and the presence of large numbers of dysplastic cells in the superficial layers of the epithelium.

The acetowhite appearance is not unique to CIN and early cancer. It is also seen in other situations when increased nuclear protein is present: for example in immature squamous metaplasia, congenital transformation zone, in healing and regenerating epithelium (associated with inflammation), leukoplakia (hyperkeratosis) and condyloma. While the acetowhite epithelium associated with CIN and preclinical early invasive cancer is more dense, thick and opaque with well demarcated margins from the surrounding normal epithelium, the acetowhitening associated with immature squamous metaplasia and regenerating epithelium is less pale, thin, often translucent, and patchily distributed without well defined margins. Acetowhitening due to inflammation and healing is usually distributed widely in the cervix, not restricted to the transformation zone. The acetowhite changes associated with immature metaplasia and inflammatory changes quickly disappear, usually within 30-60 seconds.

Acetowhitening associated with CIN and invasive cancer quickly appears and persists for more than one minute. The acetic acid effect reverses much more slowly in high-grade CIN lesions and in early pre-clinical invasive cancer than in low-grade lesions, immature metaplasia and sub-clinical HPV changes. It may last for 2-4 minutes in the case of high-grade lesions and invasive cancer.

Acetowhitening also occurs in the vagina, external anogenital skin and anal mucosa (see Table 4.2). The acetowhite reaction varies in intensity, within and between patients. The reaction is often associated with other visual signs in the same area, and is not specific for intraepithelial preneoplasia. Invasive cancer may or may not be acetowhite; it usually has other distinguishing features that will alert the colposcopist. For these reasons, practical training is necessary to develop knowledge, skills and experience in colposcopy. Learning colposcopy requires more supervised practice than most other endoscopic procedures, because of the microscopic interpretation that must occur *in vivo*, in addition to the technical aspects of the endoscopic procedure.

As previously stated, the main goal of colposcopy is to detect the presence of high-grade CIN and invasive cancer. To effectively achieve this, the entire epithelium at risk should be well visualized, abnormalities should be identified accurately and assessed for their degree of abnormality, and appropriate biopsies must be taken. The colposcopic documentation and the biopsies taken by a colposcopist are important indicators for quality management in colposcopy clinics.

Table 4.2: Preneoplastic intraepithelial lesions in the anogenital tract that show the acetowhitening reaction

Cervical intraepithelial neoplasia (CIN)

Vaginal intraepithelial neoplasia (VAIN)

Vulvar intraepithelial neoplasia (VIN)

Anal intraepithelial neoplasia (AIN)

Penile intraepithelial neoplasia (PIN)

Principles of Schiller's (Lugol's) iodine test

The principle behind the iodine test is that original and newly formed mature squamous metaplastic epithelium is glycogenated, whereas CIN and invasive cancer contain little or no glycogen. Columnar epithelium does not contain glycogen. Immature squamous metaplastic epithelium usually lacks glycogen or, occasionally, may be partially glycogenated. Iodine is glycophilic and hence the application of iodine solution results in uptake of iodine in glycogen-containing epithelium. Therefore, the normal glycogen-containing squamous epithelium stains mahogany brown or black after application of iodine. Columnar epithelium does not take up iodine and remains unstained, but may look slightly discoloured due to a thin film of iodine solution; areas of immature squamous metaplastic epithelium may remain unstained with iodine or may be only partially stained. If there is shedding (or erosion) of superficial and intermediate cell layers associated with inflammatory conditions of the squamous epithelium, these areas do not stain with iodine and remain distinctly colourless in a surrounding black or brown background. Areas of CIN and invasive cancer do not take up iodine (as they lack glycogen) and appear as thick mustard yellow or saffron-coloured areas. Areas with leukoplakia (hyperkeratosis) do not stain with iodine. Condyloma may not, or occasionally may only partially, stain with iodine. We recommend the routine use of iodine application in colposcopic practice as this may help in identifying lesions overlooked during examination with saline and acetic acid and will help in delineating the anatomical extent of abnormal areas much more clearly, thereby facilitating treatment.

Documentation of colposcopic findings

The record of colposcopic findings for each visit should be documented carefully by the colposcopists themselves, immediately after the examination. This record, which can be stored on paper or electronically, forms the backbone of any medical record system that can be used for continuing patient care and performance. An example of a colposcopy record containing the important attributes of a colposcopic assessment is shown in Appendix 1. Colposcopists or clinics can adapt this form to suit their needs; the structured format is intended to prompt the colposcopist to use quantitative data, whenever possible, and to capture qualitative data in a drawing. Colposcopists, even in the same clinic, generally record their findings in a wide variety of ways. Various experts have recommended standardized representations of colposcopic findings in a drawing; the symbolic representations suggested by René Cartier are a good example of what may be useful in this context (Cartier & Cartier, 1993).

Since an examination of the entire lower genital tract should be performed whenever a woman is referred for colposcopy, the colposcopist must be able to record the clinical findings in the vaginal, vulvar, perianal and anal epithelium. These findings can be combined with the cervical record on one page or kept on a separate page.

Chapter 5

The colposcopic examination step-by-step

- It is important to explain the examination procedure and reassure the woman before colposcopy. This will ensure that the woman relaxes during the procedure.

- Written informed consent should be obtained from the woman before the colposcopic examination.

- Relevant medical and reproductive history should be obtained before the procedure.

- A strict adherence to the essential steps involved in colposcopic examination ensures that common errors are avoided.

- It is important to visualize the squamocolumnar junction in its entire circumference, otherwise, the colposcopic procedure is termed 'unsatisfactory'.

- One should identify the transformation zone (TZ) during the colposcopic procedure. The proximal limit of the TZ is defined by the squamocolumnar junction, while the distal limit of the transformation zone is identified by finding the most distal crypt openings or nabothian follicles in the lips of the cervix and by drawing an imaginary line connecting these landmarks.

- It is essential to obtain directed biopsies, under colposcopic control, from abnormal/-suspicious areas identified.

- Colposcopy during pregnancy requires considerable experience. As pregnancy progresses, cervical biopsy is associated with increased probability and severity of bleeding, which is often difficult to control. The risk of biopsy should always be weighed against the risk of missing an early invasive cancer. Non-invasive lesions may be evaluated post-partum.

The steps involved in colposcopic examination to identify cervical neoplasia are described in detail in this chapter. A strict adherence to this examination protocol ensures that common errors in colposcopic practice are avoided to a large extent. It is advised that students should have thoroughly reviewed the anatomical and pathophysiological basis of colposcopic practice described in the previous chapters before going any further.

Practise first on inanimate objects
The colposcope can be thought of as an extension of the clinician's visual sense; as such, with practice, it should become a familiar tool rather than an impediment - a part of the colposcopist's body, so to speak. When one is learning colposcopy, it is helpful to become familiar with the equipment that one will be using. It is a good idea to practise focusing on inanimate objects (such as apples, oranges, flowers, small bottles with labels, etc.) in the examining room, using different light intensities and magnifications, with and without the green and/or blue filter.

Two adjustments may be required to personalize the instrument for use. The instrument should be adjusted to suit the interpupillary distance of the colposcopist to achieve stereoscopic vision by altering the separation between the two ocular lenses (eyepieces). The eyepieces should be kept wide open initially. If when looking through the colposcope, one can see two separate fields of vision, the eyepieces should be brought closer until the two fields merge to give a stereoscopic binocular vision. The eyepieces can also be adjusted to compensate for variation in an individual colposcopist's vision by changing the focus of each ocular lens, which can be matched to the correction required (+ or - dioptres), if any, by using the dioptre scale on the side of the eyepieces. This is achieved by looking through the right eyepiece with the left eye closed and moving the colposcope and by tuning the fine focus using the fine focus handle so that the image comes into focus. Without moving the colposcope, and closing the right eye, the left eyepiece should then be turned slowly until the image comes into focus. Now the instrument has been adjusted to suit the individual's vision. Those with normal eyesight or eyesight corrected by glass need not do any correction of dioptre setting.

One method of practising colposcopic biopsy technique on an inanimate object involves using a piece of pipe that matches the diameter and length of the vagina (about 5 cm wide and 15 cm long) and a foam rubber ball that can be cut into sections and wedged into the distal end of the pipe. Typewriter correction fluid or similar paint can be used to simulate lesions on the surface of the foam rubber. These painted lesions form the targets with which to practise colposcopy. This avoids the problem of procuring animal tissues on which to practise and the attendant problems of storing and cleaning them up. Biopsies should be done under colposcopic visualization whenever possible, so the biopsy technique should be learned using the colposcope. Whenever possible the student should be under the supervision of an instructor who is experienced in colposcopy and, if possible, has taken a training course. Interactive learning, based on actual patients, will accelerate the learning curve. In practice sessions, it is worthwhile learning to use colposcopy assessment forms (see Appendix 1) to document the findings and the location where a biopsy has been taken.

Steps in the colposcopic examination

Many authors have provided good advice about the proper way to conduct a colposcopic examination (Campion *et al.*, 1991; Cartier & Cartier, 1993; Coppleson *et al.*, 1993; Soutter 1993; Wright *et al.*,

1995; Anderson *et al.*, 1996; Burghart *et al.*, 1998; Singer & Monaghan 2000). Though there are different schools of thought and practice of colposcopy, the approach discussed in this manual is based on the classical or extended colposcopy technique.

Colposcopists often form their own judgements regarding what they believe is essential to the colposcopic examination, and discard much of what they deem not to be useful. It seems that colposcopic practice is somewhat flexible in content and the order of performance of different steps may vary in different settings, since circumstances change according to cultural and other contextual settings in which colposcopy is conducted worldwide. However, we recommend that the following steps be carefully followed during the learning phase, as well as during routine colposcopic practice. Wherever possible, we have given the reason for each step. Often the evidence for the value of each step will come with experience. The evaluation of normal and abnormal colposcopic findings is given in Chapters 6 to 9.

Explain the procedure to the woman

Women referred to a colposcopy clinic may not have had the procedure explained to them in detail before their arrival. For literate women, pamphlets on what an abnormal cervical cytology or other screening test means and an explanation of the colposcopic examination may be helpful. It is important for all women to have a prior explanation of the procedure and reassurance by the clinic nurse or the colposcopist. Colposcopic examination may prove difficult and yield suboptimal results if the woman does not relax during the procedure. Privacy during the consultation and examination is of utmost importance.

Obtain informed consent

After the procedure has been explained to the woman, written informed consent should be obtained, before colposcopy. The written consent form should include information about the colposcopic examination and the usual procedures that may accompany it, such as biopsy, endocervical curettage and photography, and summarize the usual complications (less serious and more frequent ones, as well as more serious but less frequent ones) that may occur. An example of a written informed consent form is given in Appendix 2. It may be preferable to obtain informed consent each time, if a woman requires subsequent colposcopic examinations.

Treatment for a colposcopically confirmed cervical intraepithelial neoplasia (CIN) may be planned during the same visit as colposcopy, to minimize the number of visits and to ensure compliance with treatment, as women may not be willing (for a variety of reasons) to make a subsequent visit to complete treatment. An ablative treatment like cryotherapy (see Chapter 12) may be planned after directing a biopsy during colposcopy (so that histopathology results for the treated lesion will be available at a later date). On the other hand, an excisional treatment such as loop electrosurgical excision procedure (LEEP) (see Chapter 13) will produce a tissue specimen that will help to establish the pathological nature of the lesion treated. If such an appproach to treatment immediately after colposcopy in the same visit is planned, the informed consent process should deal with treatment issues as well. The possible consequences of this approach in terms of overtreatment or unnecessary treatment, as well as the potential side-effects and complications of the treatment procedure, should be explained before obtaining the informed consent.

Obtain a relevant medical history

The woman's medical history is usually taken after her written informed consent has been obtained. Most women are referred after a screening examination and it is ideal to have the result of the screening test available at the time of colposcopic examination. If the woman has been referred because of abnormal cytology results, it is ideal to have a written copy of the previous smear(s) on hand at the time of the colposcopy appointment. Relevant obstetric and gynaecological history and history of any relevant exposures (e.g., number of pregnancies, last menstrual period, history of oral contraceptive use, hormonal supplements, sexually transmitted infections, etc.) should be obtained and recorded with the aid of a form designed for this purpose. It is important to enquire about the last menstrual period in order to assess the possibility of pregnancy or menopause.

Insert the vaginal speculum and inspect the cervix

The woman should be in a modified lithotomy position on an examining table with heel rests, or stirrups or knee crutches. It is preferable to place the buttocks slightly over the end of the table. It is important to ask the woman to relax. Positioning the buttocks in this way makes it much easier to insert the speculum and

to manipulate it in different axes, if needs be. An instrument tray with essential instruments for colposcopy is placed beside the couch (Figure 4.3). A medium-size bivalve speculum (Cusco, Grave, Collin's or Pedersen's) is usually adequate. Warm, clean water on the speculum is the preferred lubricant, as it warms the metal, but does not interfere with the interpretation of cervical specimens, such as a cytology smear. If the woman has extremely lax vaginal walls, a lateral vaginal side-wall retractor (Figure 4.5) or a latex condom on the speculum (with the tip of the condom cut 1 cm from the nipple) is helpful (Figure 4.9). Particular care should be taken to align the blades of the vaginal side-wall retractor perpendicular to the vaginal speculum to prevent vaginal pinching. The skills for this manoeuvre come with practice. In very obese women, it may be preferable to use two Sim's specula to retract the anterior and posterior vaginal walls.

Once the speculum is inserted and the blades are widely separated, a good view of the cervix and the vaginal fornices is obtained. This may also result in some eversion of the lips of the multiparous cervix, allowing the lower portion of the endocervical canal to come into view. After exposing the cervix, one should assess the nature of the cervico-vaginal secretions and note any obvious findings such as ectropion, polyp, nabothian follicles, congenital transformation zone, atrophy, inflammation and infection, leukoplakia (hyperkeratosis), condylomata, ulcer, growth and any obvious lesions in the vaginal fornices. Following this, excess mucus should be removed gently from the cervix with saline-soaked cotton swabs. Swabbing with dry cotton balls is discouraged, as these may induce traumatic bleeding and subepithelial petechiae. Loss of epithelium and bleeding due to rough and traumatic manipulation of the speculum and swabs should be avoided.

Obtain a cervical cytology smear, if necessary

It is likely that the woman has been referred because of an abnormal cytology result; it is, therefore, debatable whether a repeat smear is necessary in such instances. On the other hand, if the colposcopist is interested in the results of a repeat cytology test, the cervix should be sampled for the smear before the application of any solution, such as acetic acid. Sometimes the process of taking a smear will cause bleeding, but this usually subsides gradually after acetic acid is applied.

Obtain specimens for laboratory examination, if necessary

Any necessary swab for screening or diagnostic work-up because of suspicious signs or symptoms should be done at this stage. For example, a swab for Neisseria gonorrhoeae culture can be obtained from the endocervical canal or pus in the vaginal fornix, and a Chlamydia trachomatis specimen can be obtained from the endocervical canal after excessive mucus has been removed. If an ulcerative lesion is found on the vagina or cervix or on the external anogenital area, the colposcopist should consider the possibility of one or more sexually transmitted infections as the cause and the appropriate work up should be performed. If a sample is required to test for example for human papillomavirus (HPV), the cervical cells should be obtained before application of acetic acid.

Following this, the cervix should be inspected at low-power magnification (5x to 10x), looking for any obvious areas of abnormality (e.g., leukoplakia).

Apply normal saline solution

Normal saline is applied to the cervix with a sprayer or cotton balls and excess liquid is removed afterwards. This is not only the ideal way to conduct a preliminary inspection for surface abnormalities (e.g., leukoplakia, condylomata), but also the best way to examine the detail of cervical capillaries and surface blood vessels. The examination of the blood vessels is further aided by using the green (or blue) filter on the colposcope to enhance the contrast of the vessels, and by using higher levels of magnification (about 15x). Although some experienced colposcopists do not routinely perform an examination after saline has been applied (instead going directly to the application of acetic acid), it has been argued that an examination should be done in all cases, since the information obtained on the location of abnormal vessels can be noted and integrated with the findings from later steps, which will determine the appropriate biopsy site(s), if any. The application of acetic acid, and even Lugol's iodine solution, to the cervix can result in tissue swelling and consequent opacity. This swelling and opacity tend to obscure some of the details of the vessels in the subepithelial tissue, so it is always is best to assess the capillaries and vessels with saline before the application of any other solution.

The other important task at this step is to identify the distal and proximal borders of the transformation zone. The inner border is defined by the entire 360-degree circumference of the squamocolumnar junction. If the junction is proximal to the external os, in the canal, it requires additional effort to visualize the entire junction. Opening the blades of the vaginal speculum and using a cotton-tipped applicator to pry the anterior lip up or the posterior lip down will often allow visualization if the junction is close enough to the os. The endocervical speculum

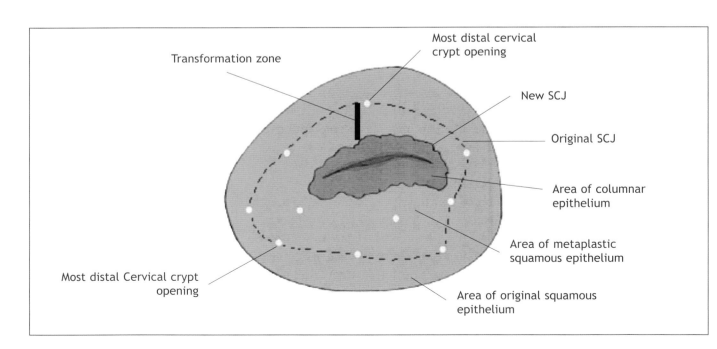

FIGURE 5.1: A method of identifying outer and inner borders of the transformation zone (SCJ: Squamocolumnar junction)

(Figure 4.6) or the lips of a long dissection forceps can also be used, and often will allow a greater length of canal to be inspected. The skill for these manoeuvres comes with practice. If the squamocolumnar junction is not visualized in its entire circumference, the colposcopic procedure is termed inadequate or unsatisfactory (see Chapter 6).

The distal limit of the transformation zone, namely the location of the original squamocolumnar junction, may be identified by finding the most distal crypt openings or nabothian follicles in the lips of the cervix and by drawing an imaginary line connecting these landmarks (Figure 5.1).

Apply acetic acid

This step may be carried out using 3-5% dilute glacial acetic acid. We prefer to use 5% dilute acetic acid as the acetowhite changes may occur faster and be more obvious than with a 3-4% solution. If white table vinegar is used, it is usually 5% acetic acid, but it is preferable to confirm the strength of the solution. The two main purposes of applying acetic acid are, first, to conduct another inspection of the entire new squamocolumnar junction and second, to detect and evaluate any areas of abnormal or atypical transformation zone (ATZ). Acetic acid should be liberally applied to the cervix with a cotton-tipped swab or cotton balls or using a 2 x 2 inches gauze or with a sprayer so that it covers the entire cervical surface, including the external os.

Wiping the cervix a few times with a cotton ball or other large applicator assists in the coagulation and removal of mucus, which in turn helps the acetic acid to penetrate to the epithelium in full strength. The mucus in the canal may be difficult to extract, but it can be easily and temporarily pushed into the os with an acetic acid-soaked cotton swab, particularly if it is obscuring the assessment of an important feature, such as the squamocolumnar junction. In the latter case, the swab also helps to apply the acid to the area of the squamocolumnar junction, which may be just inside the os, and can also be used to manipulate the cervix to view otherwise hidden areas of interest. Patience is required during this step because the acetowhitening effect of acetic acid develops gradually over the course of 60 seconds and the effect may fade afterwards. Hence, acetic acid may be reapplied every 2 to 3 minutes during the examination. A swab may be used to reapply, using the acetic acid pooled in the posterior aspect of the vagina.

Apply Lugol's iodine solution

Normal squamous (both original and mature metaplastic) epithelial cells contain stores of glycogen that give a mahogany brown or nearly black stain when an iodine-containing solution, such as Lugol's, is applied. In contrast, normal columnar epithelium does not contain glycogen and does not take up the iodine stain. Similarly, immature squamous metaplasia, inflammatory and regenerating epithelium and congenital transformation zone contain very little or no glycogen and either do not or only partially stain with iodine. Condylomata also either do not or only partially stain with iodine. Abnormal transformation zones, such as those with CIN or invasive cancer, contain very little or no glycogen. The degree of differentiation of the cells in a preneoplastic squamous lesion determines the amount of intracellular glycogen and thus the degree of staining observed. Therefore, one would expect to see a range of staining from partially brown to mustard yellow across the spectrum from low- to high-grade CIN. Usually high-grade CIN takes up less of the stain, appearing as mustard or saffron yellow areas. In the case of high-grade CIN, vigorous or repeated application of iodine may occasionally peel off the abnormal epithelium and the underlying tissue stroma may appear pale, as it lacks glycogen.

It is important always to integrate the findings of the saline, acetic acid, and iodine tests to make a colposcopic assessment. The iodine test is also very helpful for determining whether vaginal lesions are present. Application of iodine will clearly delineate the borders of a lesion before a biopsy, or treatment of the lesion, is attempted.

Perform cervical biopsies, if necessary

Once an abnormal transformation zone is detected, the area is evaluated and compared with other areas of the cervix. If any other abnormal zones are present, the colposcopist should then decide from where a biopsy or biopsies should be taken. It is essential to obtain one or more directed punch biopsies from areas colposcopically identified as abnormal and/or doubtful. Biopsy should be obtained from the area of the lesion with worst features and closest to the squamocolumnar junction. Biopsy always should be done under colposcopic control by firmly applying the biopsy instrument (Figure 4.8), with the jaws wide open (Figure 5.2), to the cervical surface to be sampled. The cervix may move back somewhat with this manoeuvre, but that is normal.

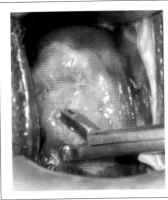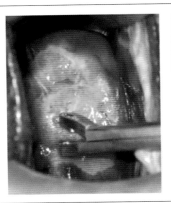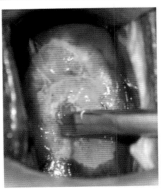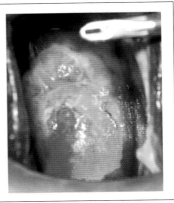

FIGURE 5.2: Biopsy technique: A toothed and sharp cutting biopsy forceps should be used for biopsy. Firmly apply the biopsy punch onto the cervix with the jaws wide open; fix the lower lip of the biopsy punch and close the jaws completely. Cutting the specimen should be carried out by quick and firm closure of the jaws. Repeated cutting and rotation of the forceps should be avoided, as this can crush the tissue sample. The removed specimen should be immediately placed in formalin. The biopsy site may be cauterized with Monsel's paste

To obtain a tissue sample, the biopsy forceps is guided under colposcopic visualization to the area from which the tissue specimen is to be obtained. The cervix may tend to slip away on pressure, but it is usually easy to grasp and remove tissue if the forceps used for biopsy has wide and sharp cutting edges, with one or two teeth to anchor the forceps while taking the biopsy (Figure 5.2). A tenaculum may be also used to fix the cervix before taking the biopsy. The jaws are then closed completely, and the specimen is removed and immediately placed in formalin. The biopsy performed should be deep enough to obtain adequate stroma, in order to exclude invasion. Cutting the specimen should be carried out by quick and firm closure of the jaws. Repeated cutting and rotation of the forceps should be avoided, as they can crush the tissue sample. The procedure is usually painless if carried out efficiently using a sharp and toothed biopsy forceps. A skin hook is sometimes useful to anchor a potential biopsy site if it is difficult to grasp with the biopsy instrument. After the biopsy has been obtained, it is advisable to indicate the site of the target area which has been biopsied, on the diagram of cervix in the reporting form. It is important to place the freshly obtained biopsy specimen in a labelled bottle containing 10% formalin. The biopsy site(s) may be cauterized with Monsel's paste or with a silver nitrate stick immediately after the procedure to control any bleeding.

Apply Monsel's paste after biopsy

It is usual practice to ensure haemostasis by applying Monsel's (ferric subsulfate) paste to the biopsy site. This is done by gently applying pressure with a cotton-tipped applicator, the tip of which has been coated with Monsel's paste (see Appendix 3). Monsel's solution is the most common haemostatic agent used after cervical biopsy or excision, and it performs well when it has a thick, toothpaste-like consistency. The paste-like consistency may be produced by exposing the stock solution to the air in a small container, which results in evaporation and thickening of the agent, or using a microwave oven. The paste-like consistency may be preserved by keeping the paste in a closed container and by adding small amount of Monsel's solution whenever it becomes dry and excessively thick.

A silver nitrate stick can also be used to cauterize a biopsy site. The haemostatic action of these chemicals is much better if the chemical is applied promptly, before bleeding begins, allowing direct contact of the chemical with the tissue rather than with blood.

Perform endocervical curettage, if necessary

There are three commonly encountered circumstances, in which an endocervical curettage (ECC) should be performed using an endocervical curette (Figure 4.7). First, if the colposcopic examination of the ectocervix has not revealed any abnormality, yet the woman has been referred because of a cytological abnormality, an ECC should be performed to properly evaluate the endocervical canal, which may contain a hidden invasive cancer or other lesion. Second, if the referral cytology indicated that a glandular lesion may be present, an ECC should be performed (regardless of the findings of the colposcopic examination). Third, an ECC should be performed if the colposcopic examination has been unsatisfactory (whether or not a cervical lesion has been detected). However, it should be mentioned that the yield of an ECC is very low in inexperienced hands, as it is frequently associated with inadequate tissue sampling. Thus, in such situations, a negative ECC should not be taken as unequivocal evidence of the absence of neoplasia in the endocervical canal.

In the above three situations, and particularly in the case of an acetowhite lesion extending into the canal, it may be prudent to excise the cervix with a cone (by LEEP or cold knife conization, as appropriate; see Chapters 11 and 13). However, this approach places a large work load on histopathology services and, as such, may not be feasible in several sub-Saharan African countries and other developing regions with extremely limited or even no histopathology services. In the assessment of women in such settings, it is left to the discretion of the colposcopist to decide whether an ECC and/or cone biopsy should be performed. Due to the risk of an adverse effect on pregnancy outcome, ECC is absolutely contraindicated in pregnant women.

Before ECC is performed, the posterior fornix must be dry to avoid the loss of curetted tissue in the acetic acid solution which accumulated during its application on the cervix. When performing ECC, the colposcopist holds the curette like a pen and scrapes the endocervical canal in firm, short, linear strokes until it has been completely sampled. During the procedure the curette should remain in the canal. When extracting the curette, care should be taken to twirl it in order to encourage the contents of the curette basket to remain trapped therein. The curettings should be put onto a piece of either gauze or brown paper, and then promptly placed into formalin. Any residual tissue can be removed from the canal with forceps. In order to avoid the potential confusion of inadvertently sampling a visible lesion on the ectocervix or including residual tissue from an ectocervical biopsy in the neighbourhood of the external os in the endocervical curette specimen, some colposcopists perform ECC under colposcopic control, before obtaining a cervical biopsy.

Inspect vaginal walls, vulva, perineum, and perianal areas

As the speculum is withdrawn, the vaginal walls and, subsequently, the vulvar, perineal, and perianal epithelium should be inspected. The surfaces are bathed with acetic acid and after one or two minutes the acetowhite areas are noted and evaluated. There is no general agreement on whether these areas should be routinely examined in this fashion, but it seems sensible, given that the examination adds very little time and effort, and that HPV has a propensity to infect these areas and cause intraepithelial lesions, most of which are treatable.

Bimanual and rectal examination

Some practitioners believe that bimanual and rectal examination should be performed before colposcopy, some believe that it should be done after, and some do not include it as a part of the normal colposcopy clinic protocol. If it is performed before colposcopy, only water should be used as a lubricant. Despite this lack of agreement, bimanual and rectal examination can provide information about the orientation of the axis of the vaginal canal before insertion of the vaginal speculum, and it allows palpation of the cervix to detect signs of nodularity or hardness and masses in other pelvic structures, such as the ovaries and uterus. It has been argued that knowledge of other abnormalities, such as sizeable uterine fibroids, can play a role in planning the best therapy for a woman.

Explain the findings to the woman

After the woman has dressed, carefully explain the examination findings and offer her the opportunity to ask questions. Review the management plan, emphasize the importance of adequate follow-up, and discuss any barriers to compliance.

Document the findings

The findings of the colposcopic examination should be recorded with the aid of appropriate forms that are filed in such a way as to be easily retrievable.

If the woman is pregnant

The effects of pregnancy on the cervix are oedema, an increase in the area of the epithelium, enlargement and opening of the os, and eversion. As pregnancy progresses, these changes are exaggerated, so that an inadequate examination at the beginning of pregnancy may become adequate by a later stage due to eversion. Certain difficulties in examination, however, become more pronounced as pregnancy progresses: the vaginal walls tend to be redundant and collapse, obscuring the view; cervical mucus is increased; increased vascularity leads to easily induced bleeding; the blood vessel pattern in cervical pseudo-decidual tissue tends to mimic invasive cancer; and CIN tends to appear as a more severe grade than it actually is (due to increased size, increased oedema and vasculature pattern). Thus considerable experience is required for colposcopy in pregnancy.

The steps in the colposcopic procedure for a pregnant woman are similar to those for a non-pregnant woman, but extra care must be taken not to injure any tissues when a digital examination or speculum insertion is performed. If a repeat cytology smear is needed, this may be performed using a spatula, by applying gentle pressure to avoid bleeding. Some may prefer to obtain a cytology sample at the end of the colposcopic procedure, in order to avoid inducing bleeding that may obscure the colposcopic field, but this may result in a poor hypocellular sample, as cells might have been washed away during the different steps of the colposcopic procedure.

As pregnancy progresses, cervical biopsy is associated with an increased probability and degree of bleeding, which may often be difficult to control. The risk of biopsy should always be weighed against the risk of missing an early invasive cancer. All lesions suspicious of invasive cancer must be biopsied or wedge excised. Sharp biopsy forceps should be used, as they will produce less tearing of tissue. Biopsy should always be carried out under colposcopic vision to control depth. The prompt application of Monsel's paste or silver nitrate to the biopsy site, immediate bed rest for 15 to 30 minutes, and the use of a tampon or other haemostatic packing to put pressure on the biopsy site are helpful to minimize bleeding. Some women may need an injection of pitressin into the cervix or suturing for haemostasis. To avoid a large amount of tissue slough, due to the effect of Monsel's paste, haemostatic packs should not be left in place for more than a few hours after the paste has been applied. Alternatively, cervical biopsy in a pregnant woman may be performed with diathermy loop. If colposcopy is inadequate, and cytology suggests invasive cancer, a conization must be performed, ideally in the second trimester. Non-invasive lesions may be evaluated post-partum.

Chapter 6

Colposcopic appearance of the normal cervix

- The squamous epithelium appears as a smooth translucent epithelium with a pinkish tinge after application of normal saline solution. The original squamous epithelium appears more pink compared to the light pink colour of the metaplastic epithelium.

- The columnar epithelium appears dark red with a grape-like or sea anemone tentacles-like or villous appearance.

- Often no vascular patterns are seen on the original squamous epithelium. Occasionally, a network of capillaries may be visible in this epithelium. Tree-like branching vessels may be observed on the newly formed metaplastic squamous epithelium.

- After the application of acetic acid, the squamous epithelium appears dull and pale in contrast to the usual pink hue; the columnar epithelium looks less dark red, with pale acetowhitening of the villi resembling a grape-like appearance.

- The vast range of colposcopic appearances associated with squamous metaplasia after the application of acetic acid presents a challenge to differentiate between these normal changes and the abnormal features associated with CIN. Squamous metaplasia may appear as a patchily distributed pale cluster or sheet-like areas or as glassy, pinkish-white membranes, with crypt openings, with tongue-like projections pointing towards the external os.

- Both the original and mature squamous metaplastic epithelium stain mahogany brown or black with Lugol's iodine solution, while columnar epithelium does not. Immature squamous metaplastic epithelium usually does not stain with iodine or may partially stain if it is partially glycogenated. In postmenopausal women, squamous epithelium may not fully stain with iodine, due to the atrophy of the epithelium.

The anatomy of the cervix is summarized in Chapter 1. The colposcopic appearances of normal squamous epithelium, columnar epithelium, squamocolumnar junction, immature and mature metaplasia and the congenital transformation zone are described in this chapter. Awareness of and ability to identify the colposcopic features of the normal cervix provide the basis for differentiating between normal and abnormal colposcopic findings.

The most important anatomical concept that a colposcopist must have is how to identify the transformation zone (see Chapter 5, Figure 5.1). This anatomical zone is where cervical intraepithelial neoplasia (CIN) and invasive cervical carcinoma arise, and, therefore, is a major focal point of the colposcopic examination. Unless the provider can adequately examine the entire transformation zone with the colposcope, the colposcopic examination is termed inadequate or unsatisfactory. This means that the squamocolumnar junction should be visible in its full length. If it is only partially seen, or not at all, part of the transformation zone is not visible. The examination is thus deemed to be inadequate or unsatisfactory for the purpose of ruling out CIN and invasive carcinoma. Even though no abnormal findings may be evident in the portion of the transformation zone that is seen, the presence of cervical neoplasia cannot be ruled out clinically in the hidden areas of the transformation zone.

The following description of the colposcopic appearance of the normal cervix begins by describing the features of the normal transformation zone.

After application of normal saline solution
Squamous epithelium

The squamous epithelium, which is seen as a translucent smooth epithelium with a pinkish tinge, should be examined in great detail in order to define the landmarks of the transformation zone. The original squamous epithelium is darker pink in colour compared with the light pink or whitish-pink colour of the metaplastic squamous epithelium. If one looks closely, it is apparent in some women that a few crypt openings, which look like tiny circular holes, are scattered over the surface of the squamous epithelium (Figures 5.1 and 6.1). In some women, alternatively, one may look for the nabothian follicles. Looking distally, away from the os towards the outer part of the ectocervix, one comes to a point where no more crypt

openings and/or nabothian follicles are apparent. An imaginary line drawn connecting the most distal crypt openings and/or nabothian follicles that one can see in the cervical lips colposcopically defines the original squamocolumnar junction (the junction between the original or native squamous epithelium and the metaplastic squamous epithelium). The original squamocolumnar junction forms the outer, distal, or caudal border of the transformation zone through its entire 360-degree circumference. Sometimes, it is the subtle colour variation between the native and metaplastic squamous epithelium that defines the original squamocolumnar junction.

The next task is to identify the proximal or inner border of the transformation zone, which is defined by the new squamocolumnar junction (the line of demarcation where the metaplastic squamous and columnar epithelia meet), throughout its entire 360-degree circumference. If the colposcopist is able to trace the entire new squamocolumnar junction successfully, the colposcopic examination is classified as adequate or satisfactory with respect to evaluation of the transformation zone (Figures 5.1 and 6.1). The new squamocolumnar junction tends to recede towards, and eventually into, the canal as a woman

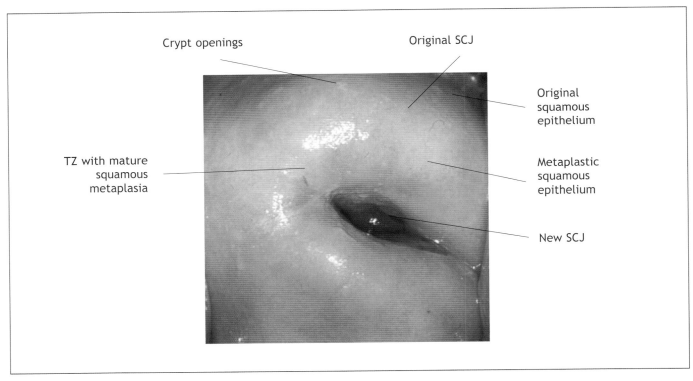

FIGURE 6.1: The entire new squamocolumnar junction (SCJ) is visible, and hence the colposcopic examination is satisfactory; the transformation zone (TZ) is fully visualized. The metaplastic squamous epithelium is pinkish-white compared to the pink original squamous epithelium

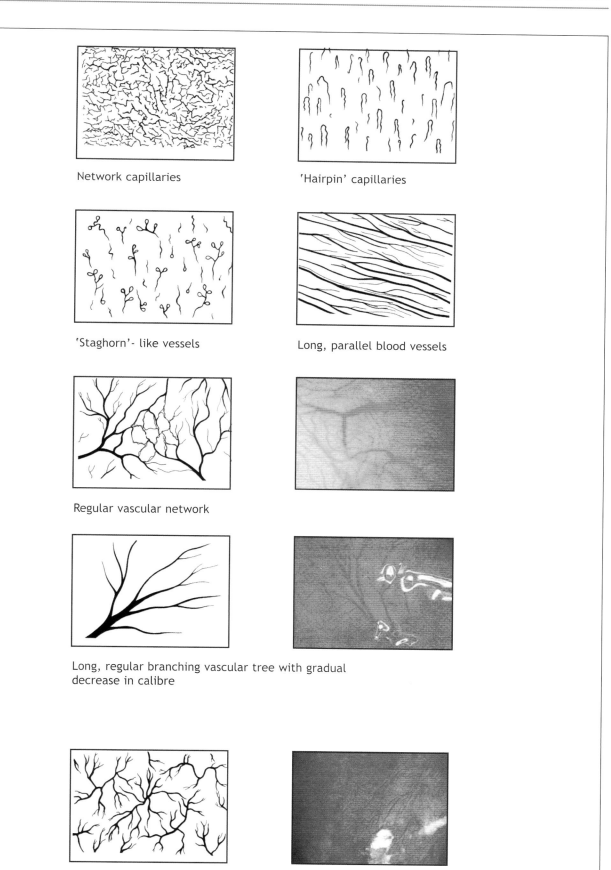

FIGURE 6.2: Normal vascular patterns

ages (Figures 1.7d, 1.7e, 1.8c and 1.8d). If the junction is proximal to the os, in the canal, it requires additional effort to visualize the entire junction. Opening the blades of the vaginal speculum and using a cotton-tipped applicator to pry the anterior lip upward or the posterior lip downward will often allow visualization of the squamocolumnar junction, if it is close enough to the os. The endocervical speculum (Figure 4.6) or the tips of a long dissection forceps also can be used, and will often allow a greater length of canal to be inspected. The skill for these manoeuvres comes with practice. The vast majority of CIN lesions occur in the transformation zone and the most severe changes tend to be closer to or abutting, rather than farther from, the new squamocolumnar junction.

Columnar epithelium

On first looking at the normal cervix in a young woman, one sees the cervical os. It usually appears to be encircled by the columnar epithelium, appearing dark red in colour with a grape-like or sea anemone tentacles-like or a villous appearance in contrast to the smooth, light pink squamous epithelium. Each columnar villous structure contains a fine capillary and the blood in the capillary and the vascularity of the underlying connective tissue give the columnar epithelium its strikingly reddish appearance. Small polyps may be detected during examination of the endocervical canal.

Vasculature

The next most important feature to observe is the vasculature. The examination of the blood vessels is facilitated by applying normal saline on the cervix and using the green (or blue) filter on the colposcope to enhance the contrast of the vessels. Use of a higher power of magnification (about 15x), if available in the colposcope, also is helpful. Depending on the thickness or opacity of the overlying squamous epithelium, smaller vessels may or may not be visible. The smaller vessels that may be visible are capillaries that are in the stroma below the epithelium.

Two types of capillaries are apparent in the native or original squamous epithelium: reticular (network) or hairpin-shaped capillaries (Figure 6.2). The reticular pattern is especially visible because the epithelium is thinner in women taking oral contraceptives and in postmenopausal women. The hairpin capillaries actually ascend vertically, loop over, and then descend back into the stroma from where they came. Since these loops are seen 'end on', the colposcopic view

usually is of dots with only a slight, if any, appearance of a loop at each. Inflammation of the cervix (e.g., trichomoniasis) often causes hairpin vessels to form staghorn-like shapes, so that the vessels become more prominent and the loop appearance is more apparent (Figure 6.2). Often no vascular pattern is seen on the original squamous epithelium.

The ectocervical vessel appearances described above are more prominent towards the outer transformation zone, nearer to the original squamocolumnar junction. In the more recently formed immature metaplastic squamous epithelium nearer the new squamocolumnar junction, other vascular patterns become more prominent. These are large (compared to capillaries) branching surface vessels with three recognizable basic patterns (Figure 6.2). The first pattern is much like a tree branching and the second is commonly seen overlying nabothian cysts (Figure 6.3). The regular structure and decrease in the calibre of the vessels towards the ends of the branches all suggest a benign (normal) nature. A third pattern sometimes occurs when healing has taken place after therapy for CIN (Figures 6.2 and 13.9): the vessels are long and run parallel to one another. The lack of other abnormal epithelial features that would suggest neoplasia is a helpful clue that the vasculature is normal. If there is any doubt, it is always prudent to take a biopsy.

The vessels in the columnar epithelium actually are terminal capillary networks. One capillary network is

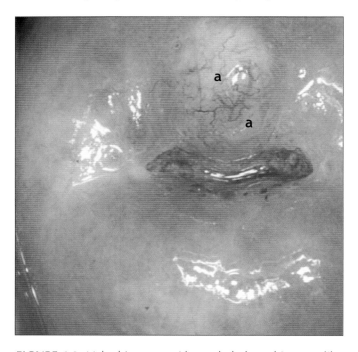

FIGURE 6.3: Nabothian cyst with regularly branching tree-like vessels (a)

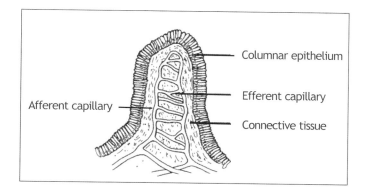

FIGURE 6.4: Capillary network in columnar villi

confined to the stromal core of each grape-like villus (Figure 6.4), which projects up to the epithelial surface. With the colposcope, the rounded tips of the individual villi are the main features seen and the top of the vessel network in each villus appears as a dot. Large, deep branching vessels may be seen in some cases.

After application of 5% acetic acid solution

Squamous epithelium

After acetic acid has been allowed to take effect (1-2 minutes), certain changes in the features seen with saline are usually apparent in the normal cervix of a young woman. The colour of the squamous epithelium tends to be somewhat dull in contrast to the usual pink hue, and the translucence is diminished so that it looks somewhat pale (Figure 6.1). In postmenopausal women the colour usually is paler than in a premenopausal woman. The landmarks and full extent of the

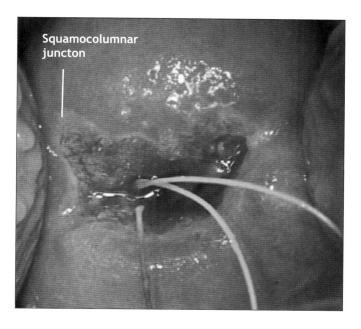

FIGURE 6.5: Prominent new squamocolumnar junction after application of 5% acetic acid

transformation zone should again be observed carefully. The squamocolumnar junction may be prominently visible as a sharp, steplike white line due to the presence of actively dividing immature squamous metaplasia around the edge, medial (proximal) to the junction (Figure 6.5). The atrophic postmenopausal squamous epithelium looks more pale, brittle, without lustre, sometimes with sub-epithelial petechiae due to the trauma to sub-epithelial capillaries resulting from the insertion of the bivalved vaginal speculum (Figure 6.6). Often the new squamocolumnar junction may not be visible in postmenopausal women as it recedes into the endocervical canal.

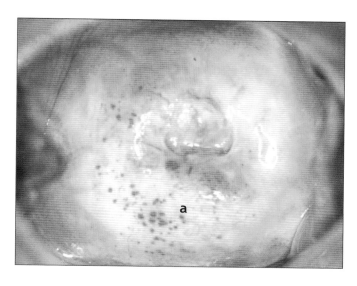

FIGURE 6.6: Postmenopausal cervix: The epithelium is pale, brittle and lacks lustre, showing sub-epithelial petechiae (a). Squamocolumnar junction is not visible

Columnar epithelium

The columnar epithelium should be inspected next. It is usually noticeably less dark red than it was with saline and the pale acetowhitening of the villi may resemble a grape-like appearance (Figure 6.7). After the endocervical mucus among the villi has been coagulated by the acetic acid and wiped away, the topography may be seen more easily. In pregnant women, the villi are hypertrophied and the grape-like appearance will be easier to observe. If a polyp is covered by the columnar epithelium (which has not yet undergone metaplastic changes), the typical grape-like appearance may be visible. More often, especially when it protrudes, the epithelium covering the polyp undergoes metaplastic changes and presents features of various stages of metaplasia.

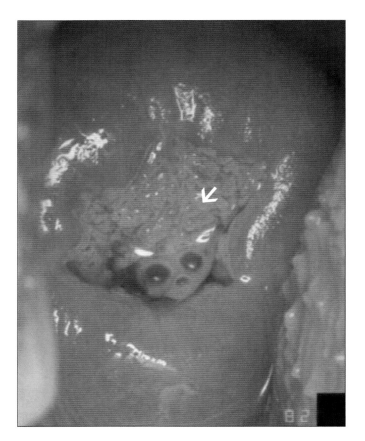

FIGURE 6.7: The colour changes in the columnar epithelium after the application of 5% acetic acid. The columnar villi turn white, obliterating the red colour of the columnar epithelium

Squamous metaplasia

During the different stages of the development of metaplasia, a vast range of colposcopic appearances may be seen. This can present a challenge to an inexperienced colposcopist, who needs to differentiate between these normal findings and the abnormal features associated with CIN. Immature metaplastic squamous epithelium that may turn mildly white after the application of acetic acid is a common source of confusion for the beginners. It is acceptable to take a biopsy when in doubt. Colposcopically, three stages of development of squamous metaplasia may be recognized (Coppleson & Reid, 1986). In the earliest stage, the translucence of the columnar epithelial villi is lost and the villi become opaque at their tips; the villi widen and flatten and successive villi fuse in clusters and sheets with a pale pink colour (Figures 6.8, 6.9 and 6.10). Consequently the metaplastic epithelium looks like a patchily distributed pale cluster, or sheet-like areas, in the ectopic columnar epithelium.

As the metaplasia progresses, the grape-like configuration of the columnar epithelium disappears and the spaces between the villi are fused with glassy, pinkish-white, finger- or tongue-like membranes pointing towards the external os (Figures 6.11 and 6.12). There may be numerous crypt openings and islands of columnar epithelium scattered throughout the metaplastic epithelium. The rims of the crypt openings may not turn white with acetic acid early in the process of metaplasia, but may turn mildly white as

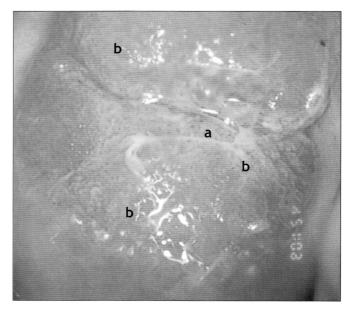

FIGURE 6.8: The earliest colposcopic changes in immature squamous metaplasia (after 5% acetic acid application) in which the tips of the columnar villi stain white (a) and adjacent villi start fusing together (b)

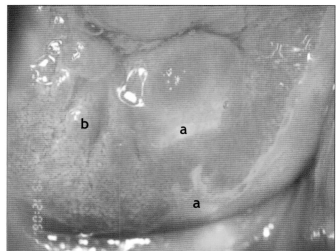

FIGURE 6.9: Immature squamous metaplasia: The columnar villi have fused together to form thin membrane (a). The adjacent villi are fusing together (b) (after 5% acetic acid application)

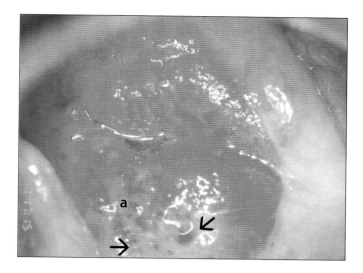

FIGURE 6.10: The glassy, pinkishwhite immature squamous metaplastic epithelium (a) with islands of columnar epithelium (narrow arrow) and crypt opening (bold arrow) (after 5% acetic acid application)

the metaplastic process progresses. Gradually, the tongue-like metaplastic areas fuse together to form a continuously advancing glassy, shining, pinkish-white or mildly pale membrane-like area (Figure 6.13).

Finally, the immature metaplastic epithelium becomes a fully developed mature metaplastic squamous epithelium resembling the original native squamous epithelium, except for the presence of some crypt openings (Figure 6.1) and nabothian retention follicles in the metaplastic epithelium (Figures 1.11,

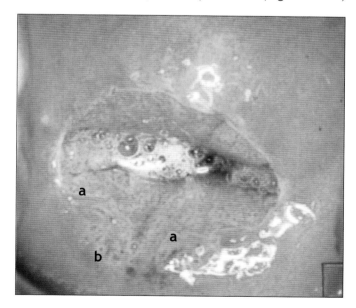

FIGURE 6.11: The prominent white line corresponds to the new squamocolumnar junction and tongues of immature squamous metaplasia (a) with crypt opening at 4-8 o'clock positions (b) (after application of 5% acetic acid)

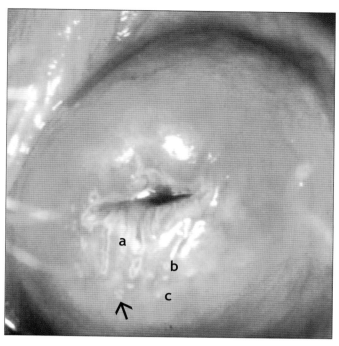

FIGURE 6.12: Appearance after 5% acetic acid application: protruding tongues (a) of immature squamous metaplasia towards the external os in the lower lip and the crypt openings (b) after application of 5% acetic acid. Some crypt openings are already covered by metaplastic epithelium (c) which may become nabothian cysts soon. Note the distal crypt opening indicated by the arrow and the pinkish white hue of the metaplastic epithelium compared to the pink colour of the original squamous epithelium

6.3 and 6.14). The retention follicles, in the beginning, may appear as white, dot-like, areas before they enlarge with progressive accumulation of mucus within the follicle, presenting as pimple- or button-like ivory-white or mildly yellowish areas (Figures 1.11, 6.3 and 6.14). The typical vessel formations in the metaplastic epithelium include long regular branching vessels with gradually decreasing calibre and a network of regular branching vessels (Figure 6.2). These vascular patterns may be seen more prominently over the nabothian follicles (Figure 6.3).

When metaplasia occurs in the epithelium covering the protruding cervical polyp, it is covered by pale white epithelium (Figure 6.15).

After application of Lugol's iodine solution

As described in the previous chapter, glycogenated cells take iodine, so that they have a uniform dark mahogany brown colour when stained with Lugol's iodine solution. Therefore, the normal vaginal and cervical squamous (both native and mature

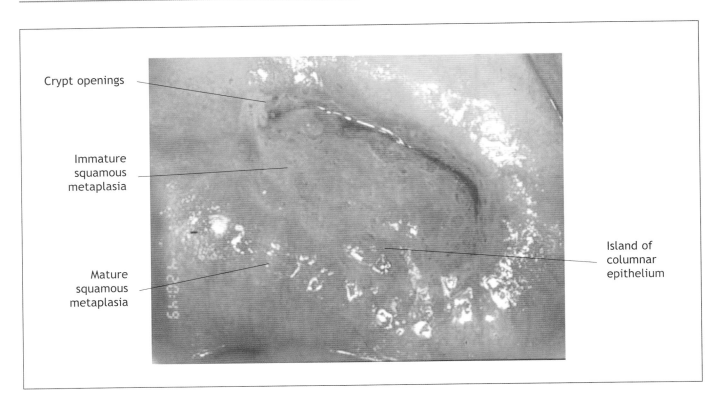

Crypt openings

Immature
squamous
metaplasia

Mature
squamous
metaplasia

Island of
columnar
epithelium

FIGURE 6.13: Pale, translucent acetowhitening due to immature squamous metaplasia with several crypt openings after application of 5% acetic acid

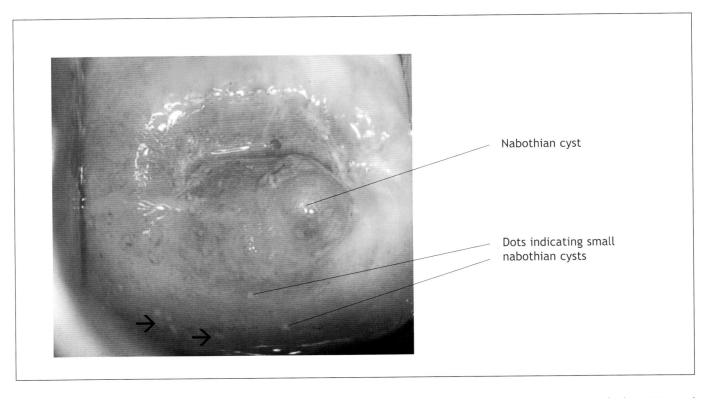

Nabothian cyst

Dots indicating small
nabothian cysts

FIGURE 6.14: Mature squamous metaplasia after the application of 5% acetic acid: Note the nabothian cyst at 5 o'clock position and the multiple dotlike areas indicating retention cysts. Narrow arrows indicate the distal crypt openings. The new squamocolumnar junction has receded into the cervical canal

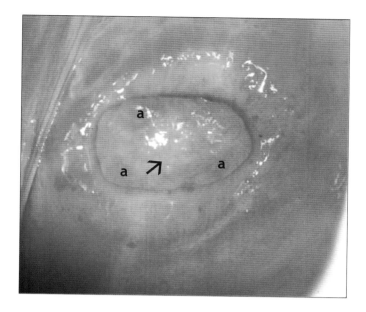

FIGURE 6.15: Immature squamous metaplastic epithelium (narrow arrow) on the polyp with intervening areas of columnar epithelium (a), after application of 5% acetic acid.

squamous metaplastic epithelium usually does not stain with iodine or may partially stain if it is partially glycogenated (Figure 6.17). The vascular features, so easily seen with saline, may be difficult to observe after application of Lugol's iodine solution. Cervical polyps do not stain with iodine, as they are usually covered with columnar or immature metaplastic epithelium (Figure 6.18). If the maturation of the metaplastic epithelium varies, one may observe various fields of no uptake or partial to full iodine uptake on the polyp. In postmenopausal women, the ectocervix may not stain fully with iodine, due to atrophy of the epithelium.

Congenital transformation zone

The congenital transformation zone stains white after application of acetic acid. In this condition, the metaplastic epithelium formed during the latter portion of fetal life, lying distal to the transformation zone formed after birth, is located far out on the ectocervix, some distance from the cervical os and, in some cases, may even extend onto the vagina. It is important to recognize this as a normal condition for which no treatment is necessary.

With acetic acid, the congenital transformation zone will usually take on a mild acetowhite stain and the capillary vasculature may have a fine mosaic pattern

metaplastic) epithelium in women in the reproductive age group will take up the stain and become mahogany brown or black (Figure 6.16). This is helpful in distinguishing normal from abnormal areas in the transformation zone that have shown faint acetowhitening. The columnar epithelium does not stain with iodine (Figure 6.16). The immature

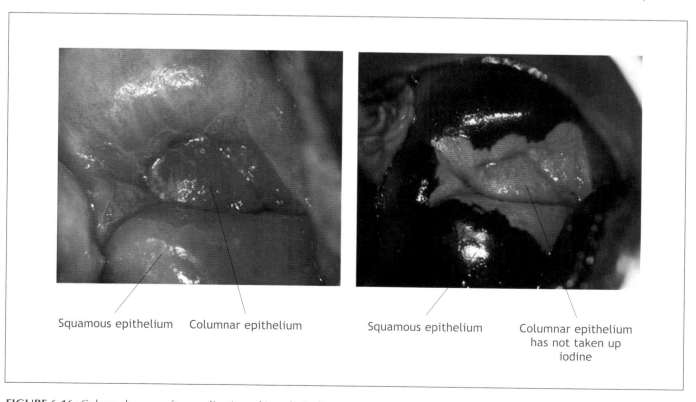

Squamous epithelium   Columnar epithelium

Squamous epithelium   Columnar epithelium has not taken up iodine

FIGURE 6.16: Colour changes after application of Lugol's iodine

53

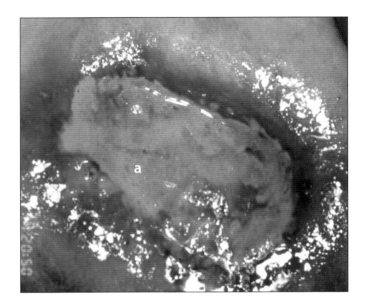

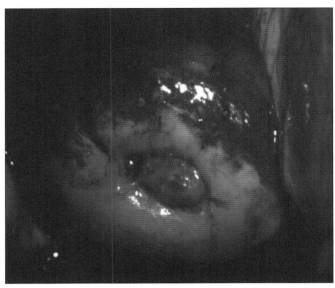

FIGURE 6.17: An area of no or partial iodine uptake in the immature squamous epithelium (a) (appearance after acetic acid application is shown in figure 6.13)

FIGURE 6.18: After application of Lugol's iodine solution, the endocervical polyp and the immature squamous metaplasia surrounding the os partially take up iodine

(see Chapter 7). It does not take up iodine after application of Lugol's iodine solution. If a biopsy is taken of the tissue to confirm the diagnosis, it is best to alert the pathologist of the colposcopic diagnosis. We emphasize that it is always necessary to provide the detailed colposcopic findings to the pathologist.

Chapter 7

Colposcopic assessment of cervical intraepithelial neoplasia

- The colposcopic diagnosis of cervical neoplasia depends on the recognition of four main features: intensity (colour tone) of acetowhitening, margins and surface contour of acetowhite areas, vascular features and colour changes after iodine application.

- The occurrence of abnormal features in a localised area in the transformation zone increases the probability of diagnosis of a neoplastic lesion.

- Considerable skill may be required to differentiate between low-grade CIN, immature squamous metaplasia and inflammatory lesions.

- Biopsy should be directed whenever in doubt.

- The observation of well-demarcated, dense, opaque, acetowhite area(s) in the transformation zone close to or abutting the squamocolumnar junction is the hallmark of colposcopic diagnosis of CIN.

- Low-grade CIN is often seen as thin, smooth acetowhite lesions with well-demarcated, but irregular, feathery or digitating or angular margins.

- High-grade CIN are associated with thick, dense, dull, opaque or greyish-white acetowhite areas with well-demarcated, regular margins, which sometimes may be raised and rolled out. They may be more extensive and complex lesions extending into the endocervical canal. The surface contour of the acetowhite areas associated with high-grade CIN lesions tend to be less smooth, or irregular and nodular. Visualization of one or more borders within an acetowhite lesion or an acetowhite lesion with varying colour intensity is associated with high-grade lesions.

- Abnormal vascular features such as punctation and mosaics are significant only if these are seen confined to acetowhite areas.

- Vascular features, such as fine punctation and/or fine mosaics in acetowhite areas, may be associated with low-grade CIN.

- Coarse punctation and/or coarse mosaics in acetowhite areas tend to occur in high-grade lesions.

- CIN lesions do not contain glycogen and thus do not stain with iodine and remain mustard or saffron yellow areas.

- Using a scoring system such as Reid's colposcopic index may guide colposcopic interpretation and diagnosis.

The colposcopic diagnosis of cervical neoplasia requires an understanding and recognition of four main features: colour tone and intensity of acetowhitening, margins and surface contour of acetowhite areas, vascular pattern and iodine staining. Colposcopy with directed biopsy is described as the reference investigation or 'gold standard' for the diagnosis of cervical precancer (Singer & Monaghan, 2000). Colposcopy has a reported sensitivity ranging from 87% to 99% to diagnose cervical neoplasia, but its specificity is lower, between 23% and 87% (Mitchell *et al.*, 1998; Belinson *et al.*, 2001).

The colposcopic features of cervical intraepithelial neoplasia (CIN) are described in this chapter to equip the student with the skills to distinguish the colposcopic findings associated with high-grade CIN (CIN 2-3) from those of low-grade lesions (CIN 1). Although the appearance of a single abnormal feature alone is not a strong indicator that a lesion is present, the occurrence of abnormal features together in a localized area in the transformation zone increases the probability of a lesion. It will become obvious during colposcopic practice that considerable skills are required to differentiate between low-grade lesions, immature squamous metaplasia and certain inflammatory conditions. The student is encouraged to obtain biopsies whenever in doubt, and to review the histopathological findings with the pathologist. Close collaboration with pathologists is obligatory and useful in improving one's diagnostic skills. At the end of this

chapter, a system that enables the colposcopist to score abnormalities is presented. This system is useful as a basis for the choice of which area(s) to select for biopsy. It is essential to biopsy the 'worst' area(s) - that is, the area(s) with the most severe changes in features.

The colposcopic findings of an abnormal or atypical transformation zone can involve the whole transformation zone but more commonly affect only a portion of it and there may be multiple distinct lesions. There is usually a distinct demarcation between normal and abnormal epithelium.

The colposcopic features that differentiate an abnormal transformation zone from the normal include the following: colour tone of acetowhite areas; surface pattern of acetowhite areas; borderline between acetowhite areas and the rest of the epithelium; vascular features and colour changes after application of iodine.

After application of normal saline solution

Following application of saline, abnormal epithelium may appear much darker than the normal epithelium.

Vasculature

Using the green (or blue) filter and higher-power magnification when necessary, the best opportunity to evaluate any abnormal vasculature patterns is before the application of acetic acid, the effect of which may obscure some or all of the changes, especially in an

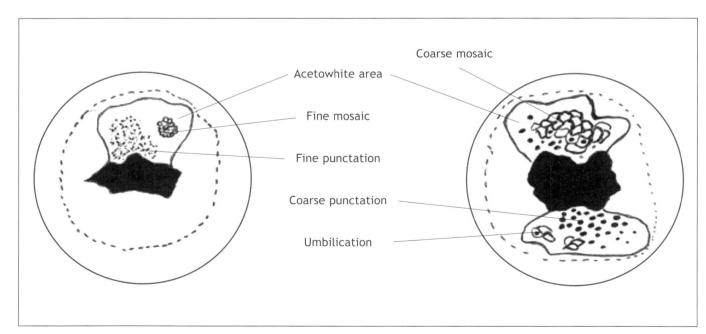

FIGURE 7.1: A schematic representation of punctation and mosaics

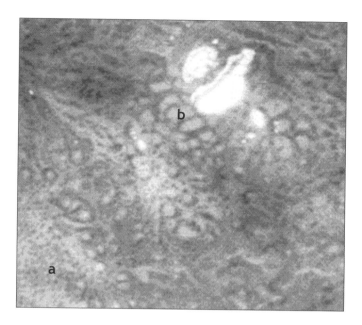

FIGURE 7.2a: Fine punctation (a) and coarse mosaic (b) seen after application of normal saline

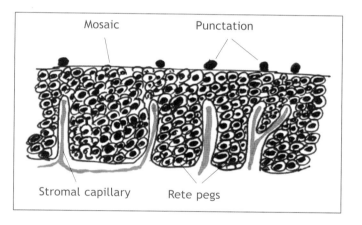

FIGURE 7.2b: Schematic diagram to show the rete pegs and the stromal capillaries which on end-on view appear as punctations

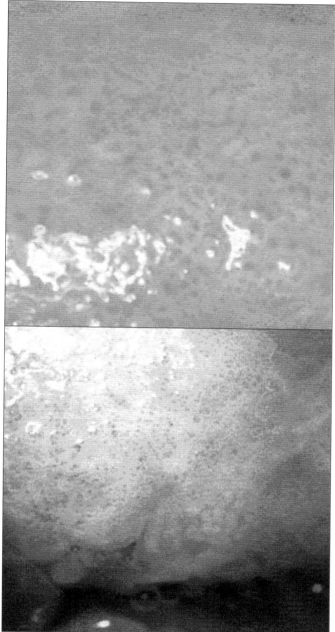

FIGURE 7.3: Coarse punctation before and after application of acetic acid

acetowhite area. The abnormalities of interest are punctation, mosaics and atypical vessels.

Capillaries: The afferent and efferent capillaries within the villi (Figure 6.4) of columnar epithelium become compressed during the normal metaplastic process and are not incorporated within the newly formed squamous epithelium. Instead, they form a fine network below the basement membrane. When CIN develops as a result of HPV infection and atypical metaplasia, the afferent and efferent capillary system may be trapped (incorporated) into the diseased dysplastic epithelium through several elongated stromal papillae (Figures 2.3 and 2.4), and a thin layer of epithelium may remain on top of these vessels. This forms the basis of the punctate and mosaic blood vessel patterns (Figures 7.1, 7.2 and 7.3). The terminating vessels in the stromal papillae underlying the thin epithelium appear as black points in a stippling pattern in an end-on view under the colposcope, making what are called punctate areas (Figures 7.1, 7.2 and 7.3). The inter-connecting blood vessels in the stromal papillae surrounding the rete pegs of the epithelium, running parallel to the surface, are observed colposcopically as cobbled areas of mosaic pattern (Figures 7.1 and 7.2). In mosaic areas, the epithelium appears as individual small, large, round, polygonal, regular or irregular blocks. Punctation and mosaic areas may be classified as either fine or coarse. Coarse changes tend to be associated with more severe degrees of abnormality. When both punctation and mosaic patterns are found to coexist, the same evaluation criteria for colposcopic prediction of disease are used as when they exist separately.

Vessels exhibiting punctation and mosaics are usually more strikingly obvious than the normal stromal vessels because these vessels penetrate into the epithelium and are thus closer to the surface. When acetic acid is applied, these abnormal vascular patterns seen to be confined to the acetowhite areas.

Fine punctation refers to looped capillaries - viewed end-on - that appear to be of fine calibre and located close to one another, producing a delicate stippling effect (Figures 7.1 and 7.2a). *Fine mosaics* are a network of fine-calibre blood vessels that appear in close proximity to one another, as a mosaic pattern, when viewed with the colposcope (Figure 7.1). These two vascular appearances may occur together and may be found in low-grade (CIN 1) lesions. The patterns do not necessarily appear throughout the whole lesion.

Coarse punctation (Figure 7.3) and *coarse mosaics* (Figures 7.1 and 7.2) are formed by vessels having larger calibre and larger intercapillary distances, in contrast to the corresponding fine changes. Coarse punctation and mosaicism tend to occur in more severe neoplastic lesions such as CIN 2, CIN 3 lesions and early preclinical invasive cancer. Sometimes, the two patterns are superimposed in an area so that the capillary loops occur in the centre of each mosaic 'tile'. This appearance is called umbilication (Figure 7.1).

Leukoplakia (hyperkeratosis)

Leukoplakia or hyperkeratosis (Figure 7.4) is a white, well-demarcated area on the cervix that may be apparent to the unaided eye, before the application of acetic acid. The white colour is due to the presence of keratin and is an important observation. Usually leukoplakia is idiopathic, but it may also be caused by chronic foreign body irritation, HPV infection or squamous neoplasia. No matter where the area of leukoplakia is located on the cervix, it should be biopsied to rule out high-grade CIN or malignancy. It is not usually possible to colposcopically evaluate the vasculature beneath such an area.

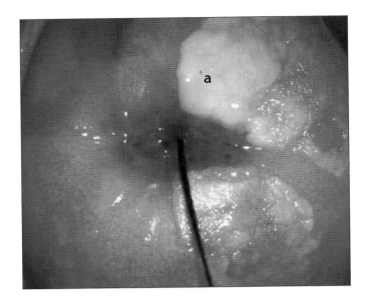

FIGURE 7.4: Hyperkeratosis (leukoplakia) (a)

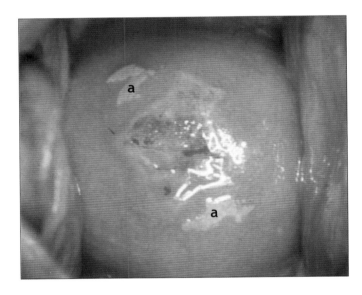

FIGURE 7.5: The geographic satellite lesions (a) far away from the squamocolumnar junction suggestive of condyloma

Condylomata

An exophytic lesion on the cervix usually represents and exhibits the characteristic features of a condyloma (Figures 7.5- 7.8). Condylomata are multiple, exophytic lesions, that are infrequently found on the cervix, but more commonly in the vagina or on the vulva. Depending on their size, they may be obvious to the naked eye. They present as soft pink or white vascular growths with multiple, fine, finger-like projections on the surface, before the application of acetic acid. Under the colposcope, condylomata have a typical appearance, with a vascular papilliferous or frond-like surface, each element of which contains a central

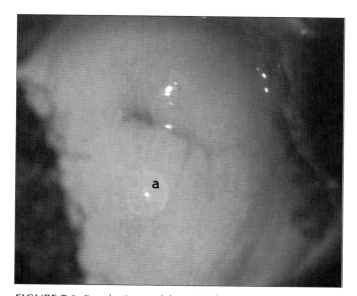
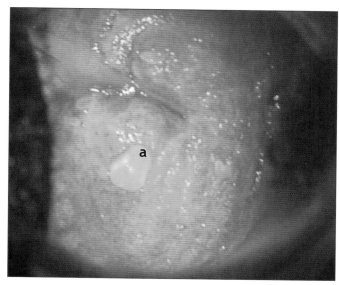

FIGURE 7.6: Exophytic condyloma in the posterior lip of the cervix (a) before and after 5% acetic acid application

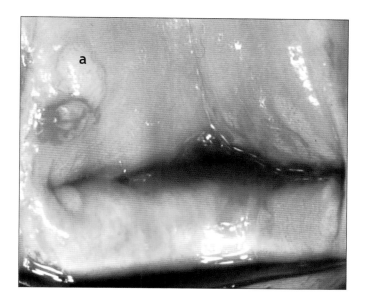
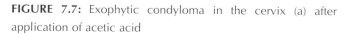
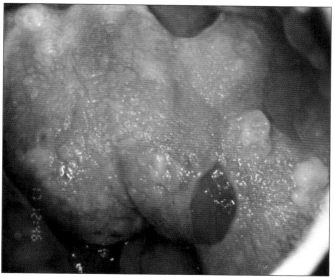

FIGURE 7.7: Exophytic condyloma in the cervix (a) after application of acetic acid

FIGURE 7.8: Condyloma with an encephaloid (cerebriform) pattern

capillary. Occasionally, the surface of a condyloma may have a whorled, heaped-up appearance with a brain-like texture, known as an encephaloid pattern (Figure 7.8). Often, the surface of the lesion may be densely hyperplastic. These lesions may be located within, but are more often found outside the transformation zone. After application of acetic acid, there is blanching of the surface with acetowhite change persisting for some time. A condyloma at the squamocolumnar junction can sometimes be confused with a prominent area of columnar epithelial villi. Both tend to be acetowhite, but condyloma is whiter. It is always prudent to obtain a biopsy to confirm the diagnosis of any exophytic lesion

and to rule out malignancy. Condylomatous lesions may not take up iodine stain or may stain only partially brown.

After the application of 5% acetic acid solution

The observation of a well demarcated, dense, opaque, acetowhite area closer to or abutting the squamocolumnar junction in the transformation zone after application of 5% acetic acid is critical. In fact, it is the most important of all colposcopic signs, and is the hallmark of colposcopic diagnosis of cervical neoplasia. The degree to which the epithelium takes up the acetic acid stain is correlated with the colour tone or intensity, the surface shine, and the duration of the effect, and, in turn, with the degree of neoplastic change in the lesion. Higher-grade lesions are more likely to turn dense white rapidly. Abnormal vascular features such as punctation, mosaicism and atypical vessels are significant only if these are seen in acetowhite areas.

The acetic acid dehydrates cells and reversibly coagulates the nuclear proteins. Thus, areas of increased nuclear activity and DNA content exhibit the most dramatic colour change. The most pronounced effects are observed in high-grade lesions and invasive cancer. A direct correlation exists between the intensity of the dull, white colour and the severity of the lesion. Less differentiated areas are associated with an intensely opaque, dull-white appearance of lesions in the transformation zone.

Flat condyloma and low-grade CIN may uncommonly present as thin, satellite acetowhite lesions detached (far away) from the squamocolumnar junction with geographical patterns (resembling geographical regions) and with irregular, angular or digitating or feathery margins (Figures 7.9- 7.13). Many low-grade CIN lesions reveal less dense, less extensive and less complex acetowhite areas close to or abutting the squamocolumnar junction with well demarcated, but irregular, feathery or digitating margins (Figures 7.10-7.16) compared with high-grade CIN lesions (Figures 7.17-7.27). High-grade lesions show well demarcated, regular margins, which may sometimes have raised and rolled out edges (Figures 7.25 and 7.26). High-grade lesions like CIN 2 or CIN 3 have a thick or dense, dull, chalk-white or greyish-white appearance (Figures 7.17-7.27). They may be more extensive and complex lesions

Table 7.1: Surface extent of acetowhite areas associated with cervical neoplasia

Cervical neoplasia	Cases	One lip of cervix (%)	Both lips (%)
CIN 1	27	21 (78)	6 (22)
CIN 2	30	17 (57)	13 (43)
CIN 3	87	36 (41)	51 (59)
Early invasive cancer	66	10 (15)	56 (85)

Adapted from Burghart *et al.*, 1998

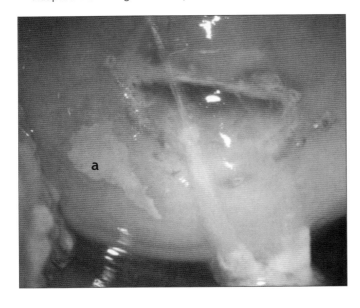

FIGURE 7.9: Geographic satellite lesion after application of 5% acetic acid (a) far away from the squamocolumnar junction, suggestive of low-grade lesion

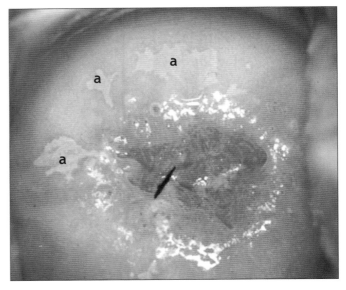

FIGURE 7.10: Geographic satellite lesions after application of 5% acetic acid (a) far away from the squamocolumnar junction, suggestive of low-grade lesions

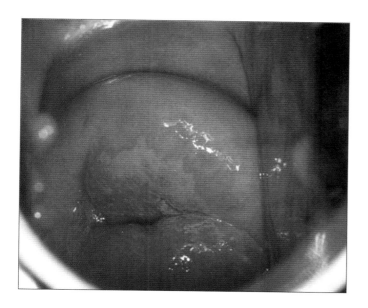

FIGURE 7.11: Thin acetowhite lesion with geographic margins in the upper lip. Histology indicated CIN 1

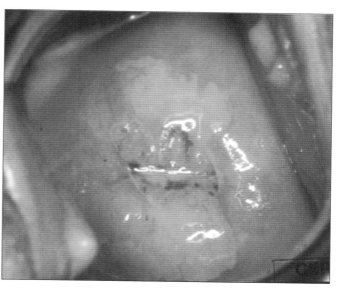

FIGURE 7.13: Mildly dense acetowhite lesions arising from the squamocolumnar junction in 12 and 6 o'clock position with irregular geographical margins, which on histology proved to be CIN 1 lesion

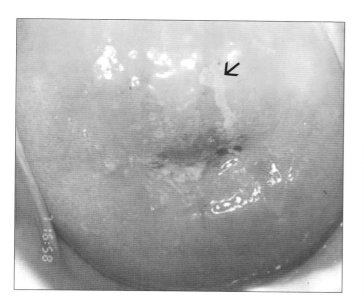

FIGURE 7.12: Mildly dense, thin, elongated acetowhite lesion with regular margins abutting the squamocolumnar junction. Note the fine mosaic at the distal end of the lesion. Histology indicated CIN 1

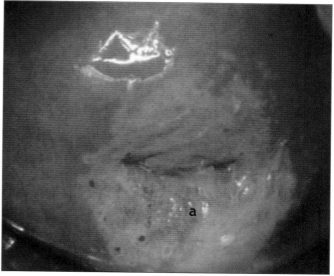

FIGURE 7.14: Note the circumorificial acetowhite CIN 1 lesion with irregular margin and fine mosaics (a)

extending into the endocervical canal (Figures 7.22-7.27) compared with low-grade lesions. High-grade lesions often tend to involve both the lips (Burghardt *et al.*, 1998) (Table 7.1). Severe or early malignant lesions may obliterate the external os (Figures 7.22 and 7.25).

As lesions become more severe, their surfaces tend to be less smooth and less reflective of light, as in

normal squamous epithelium. The surfaces can become irregular, elevated and nodular relative to the surrounding epithelium (Figures 7.20 and 7.23-7.27).

The line of demarcation between normal and abnormal areas in the transformation zone is sharp and well delineated. High-grade lesions tend to have regular, sharper borders (Figures 7.17, 7.18, 7.19, 7.21,

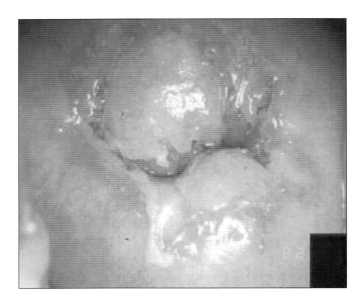

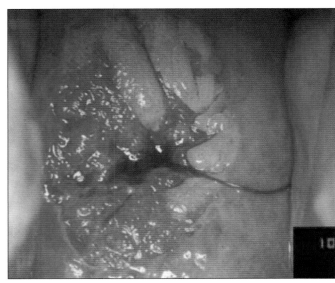

FIGURE 7.15: Moderately dense acetowhite lesions with irregular margins in the anterior and posterior lips (CIN 1)

FIGURE 7.17: Moderately dense acetowhite lesions with well defined margins and coarse punctations in the anterior lip and in 3 o'clock position (CIN 2 lesion)

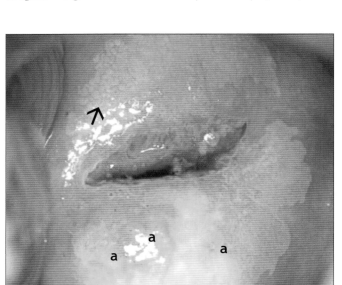

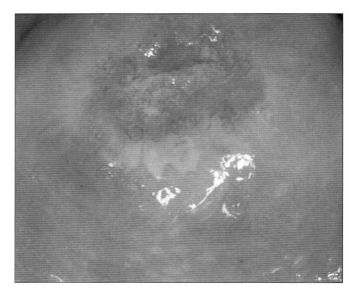

FIGURE 7.16: Circumorificial, mild to dense acetowhite lesion with fine mosaic (arrow). Histology indicated CIN 1. Note the internal borders within the lesion (a)

FIGURE 7.18: Dense, well defined acetowhite area with regular margins and coarse mosaic (CIN 2 lesion)

7.23, 7.25 and 7.26) than low-grade lesions (Figures 7.13-7.16). Visualization of one or more borders within an acetowhite lesion ('lesion within lesion') (Figure 7.21) or a lesion with differing colour intensity (Figure 7.16) is an important observation indicating neoplastic lesions, particularly high-grade lesions. The crypt openings that are involved in high-grade precursor lesions may have thick, dense and wide acetowhite rims called cuffed crypt openings (Figure 7.26). These are whiter and wider than the mild, line-like acetowhite rings that are sometimes seen around normal crypt openings.

The cardinal features that should differentiate between the CIN lesions and immature metaplasia are the less dense and translucent nature of the acetowhitening associated with metaplasia, and the

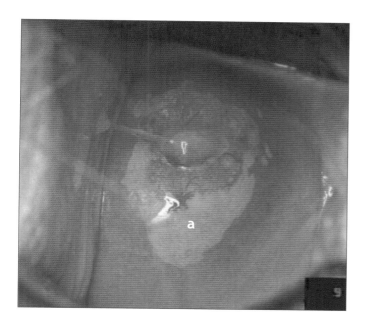

FIGURE 7.19: A dense acetowhite lesion with varying colour intensity and coarse mosaics (a) in a CIN 2 lesion

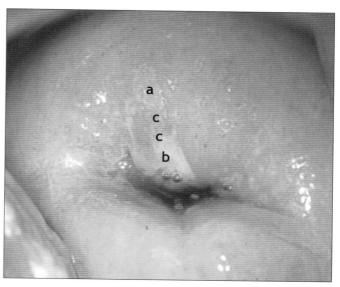

FIGURE 7.21: An acetowhite lesion arising at 12 o'clock position, abutting the squamocolumnar junction. Note the two colour intensities in the same lesion (a and b) with an internal border within the same lesion (c). This is an example of a lesion within a lesion

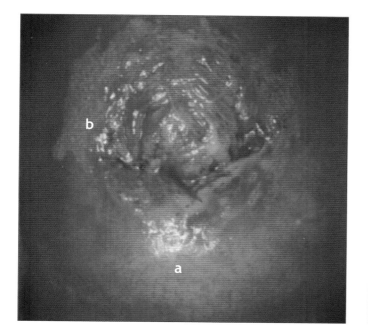

FIGURE 7.20: Acetowhite lesions with coarse punctation (a) and mosaics (b) in a CIN 2 lesion

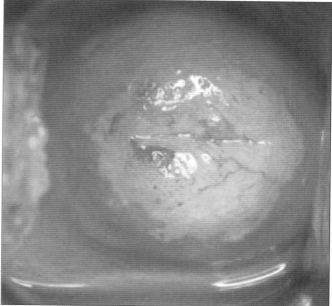

FIGURE 7.22: A circumorificial dense opaque acetowhite area with coarse mosaics (CIN 3 lesion)

lack of a distinct margin between the acetowhite areas of immature metaplasia and the normal epithelium. The line of demarcation between normal epithelium and acetowhite areas of metaplasia in the transformation zone is diffuse and invariably blends

with the rest of the epithelium (Figures 6.8-6.13). The finger-like or tongue-like projections of the metaplastic epithelium often point towards the external os centripetally (Figures 6.11 and 6.12). The acetowhite lesions associated with CIN are invariably

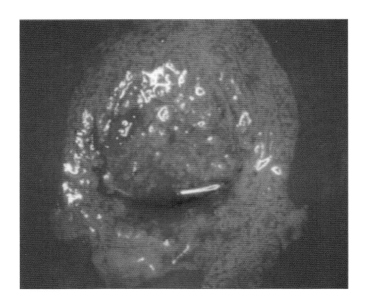

FIGURE 7.23: A dense acetowhite lesion with regular margin and coarse, irregular punctation in a CIN 3 lesion

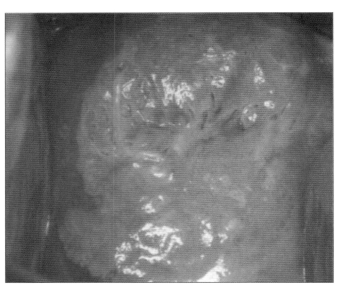

FIGURE 7.25: Note the intensely dense, complex, acetowhite lesion (CIN 3 lesion) with raised and rolled out margins, obliterating the external os

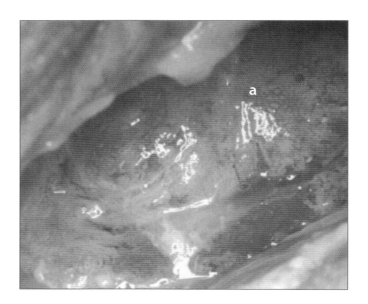

FIGURE 7.24: Coarse mosaics (a) in a CIN 3 lesion

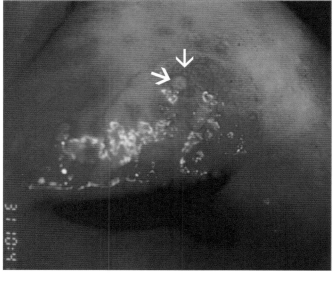

FIGURE 7.26: A dense acetowhite lesion with raised and rolled out margins with a cuffed crypt opening (dense arrow) and coarse mosaics with umblication, suggestive of a CIN 3 lesion

located in the transformation zone closer to or abutting, and appearing to arise from, the squamocolumnar junction (Figures 7.11-7.21). They spread centrifugally, pointing away from the external os. The line of demarcation between normal squamous epithelium, inflammatory lesions, and regenerating epithelium is also diffuse (Figures 9.2 and 9.5).

To summarize, acetowhite staining is not specific for CIN and may also occur, to some extent, in areas of immature squamous metaplasia, the congenital transformation zone, inflammation and healing and regenerative epithelium. However, acetowhite changes associated with CIN are found localized in the transformation zone, abutting the squamocolumnar

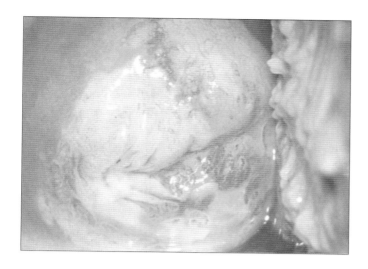

FIGURE 7.27: A dense acetowhite, opaque, complex, circumorificial CIN 3 lesion

junction and well demarcated from the surrounding epithelium. Low-grade lesions tend to be thin, less dense, less extensive, with irregular, feathery, geographic or angular margins and with fine punctation and/or mosaic; sometimes, low-grade lesions may be detached from the squamocolumnar junction; and atypical vessels are seldom observed in low-grade lesions. On the other hand, high-grade lesions are associated with dense, opaque, grey white, acetowhite areas with coarse punctation and/or mosaic and with regular and well demarcated borders; these lesions often involve both lips and may occasionally

harbour atypical vessels; CIN 3 lesions tend to be complex, involving the os.

After application of Lugol's iodine solution

Lugol's iodine solution is abundantly applied with a cotton swab to the whole of the cervix and visible parts of the vagina. The periphery of the cervix, fornices and vaginal walls must be observed until the epithelium is strongly stained dark brown or almost black by iodine. Normal vaginal and cervical squamous epithelium and mature metaplastic epithelium contain glycogen-rich cells, and thus take up the iodine stain and turn black or brown. Dysplastic epithelium contains little or no glycogen, and thus does not stain with iodine and remains mustard or saffron yellow (Figures 7.28-7.32). This colour difference is helpful in distinguishing normal from abnormal areas in the transformation zone that have shown faint acetowhitening. Columnar epithelium does not stain with iodine and immature metaplasia only partially stains, if at all. Atrophic epithelium also stains partially with iodine and this makes interpretation difficult in post menopausal women. Condylomatous lesions also do not, or only partially, stain with iodine (Figure 7.33).

Atypical epithelium of CIN may be less firmly attached to the underlying stroma, from which it may easily detach or peel off, after repeated application with different solutions, resulting in a true erosion (epithelial defect) exposing the stroma. Such true

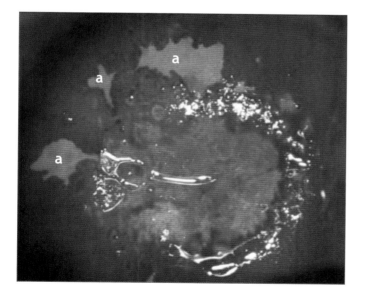

FIGURE 7.28: Satellite lesions (a) do not stain with iodine after the application of Lugol's iodine solution and remain as thin yellow areas (see the appearance after acetic acid application in Figure 7.10)

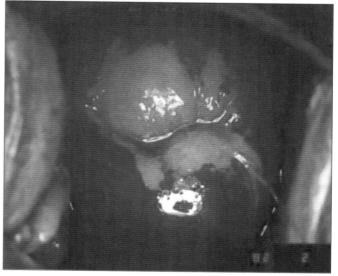

FIGURE 7.29: A CIN 1 lesion with a mustard yellow iodine-negative area with irregular margins (see the appearance after acetic acid application in Figure 7.15)

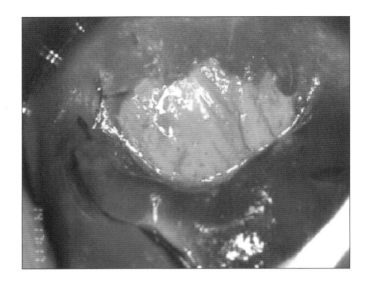

FIGURE 7.30: Mustard yellow iodine-negative area in the anterior lip (CIN 2 lesion) after the application of Lugol's iodine solution

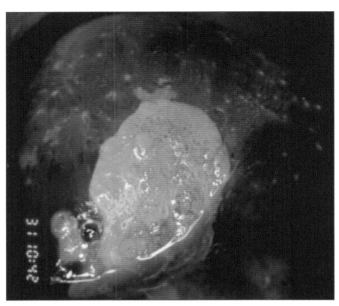

FIGURE 7.32: A dense mustard yellow iodine-negative area in the upper lip suggestive of CIN 3 lesion (see the appearance after acetic acid application in Figure 7.26)

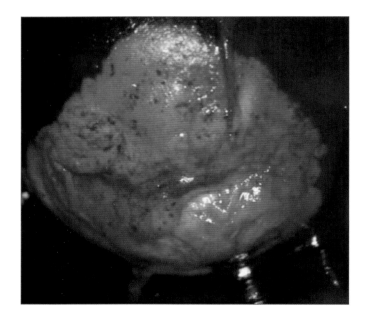

FIGURE 7.31: Dense saffron yellow iodine-negative area of a CIN 3 lesion after the application of Lugol's iodine solution. Note the surface irregularity.

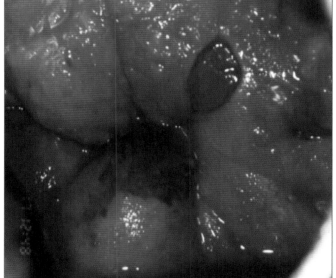

FIGURE 7.33: A condylomatous lesion does not stain with iodine (see the appearance after acetic acid application in Figure 7.8)

erosions may easily be observed after iodine application, as the stroma does not stain with iodine.

Determining the nature of the lesion

The colposcopic detection of CIN essentially involves recognizing the following characteristics: the colour tone, margin and surface contour of the acetowhite epithelium in the transformation zone, as well as the arrangement of the terminal vascular bed and iodine staining. Variations in quality and quantity of the above atypical appearances help in differentiating CIN from physiological, benign, infective, inflammatory and reactive changes in the cervix. Grading schemes, based on these variations may guide the colposcopic diagnosis.

Table 7.2: Modified Reid colposcopic index

Feature	0 points	1 point	2 points
Colour of acetowhite (AW) area	Low-intensity acetowhitening; snow-white, shiny AW; indistinct AW; transparent AW; AW beyond the transformation zone	Grey-white AW with shiny surface	Dull, oyster-white; Grey
AW lesion margin and surface configuration	Feathered margins; angular, jagged lesions; flat lesions with indistinct margins; microcondylomatous or micropapillary surface	Regular lesions with smooth, straight outlines	Rolled, peeling edges; internal demarcations (a central area of high-grade change and peripheral area of low-grade change)
Vessels	Fine/uniform vessels; poorly formed patterns of fine punctuations and/or fine mosaic; vessels beyond the margin of transformation zone; fine vessels within microcondylomatous or micropapillary lesions	Absent vessels	Well defined coarse punctation or coarse mosaic
Iodine staining	Positive iodine uptake giving mahogany brown colour; negative uptake of lesions scoring 3 points or less on above three categories	Partial iodine up-take by a lesion scoring 4 or more points on above three categories – variegated, speckled appearance	Negative iodine uptake by a lesion scoring 4 or more points on the above three criteria

Scoring: A score of 0 to 2 points = Likely to be CIN 1; 3-4 points = Overlapping lesion: likely to be CIN 1 - 2; 5 to 8 points = Likely to be CIN 2 - 3 lesions.

Table 7.3: Grading abnormal colposcopic findings using two categories

Grade	Findings
1. Insignificant	The acetowhite epithelium is usually shiny or semitransparent. The borders are not sharp, with or without fine-calibre vessels (fine punctation and/or fine mosaic), which have ill-defined patterns and short intercapillary distances. There is an absence of atypical vessels.
2. Significant	Dense acetowhite or grey opaque epithelium is sharply bordered. There are dilated calibre, irregular shaped or coiled vessels (coarse punctation and/or mosaic). Atypical vessels and sometimes irregular surface contour indicate either imminent or invasive cancer.

Adapted from Coppleson *et al.*, 1993 b

We recommend that the student should become familiar with the current colposcopic terminology given in Appendix 4 and use this to record the colposcopic findings (Stafl & Wilbanks, 1991).

The colposcopist is also encouraged to make a colposcopic prediction (or 'diagnosis') at the end of the colposcopic session in terms of normal (or negative), low-grade CIN, high-grade CIN, invasive cancer, other (e.g., inflammation etc.) and unsatisfactory colposcopy. Use of a scoring or grading system may guide colposcopic interpretation and diagnosis in a less subjective manner and helps developing a systematic approach to colposcopy. The modified Reid colposcopic score (Table 7.2 and Appendix 5) based on the colposcopic index proposed by Reid & Scalzi (1985) is quite useful for this purpose. We recommend that beginners routinely use this scoring system to decide whether or not a lesion is CIN and to select biopsy sites. An alternative may be a two-class grading system developed by Coppleson et al (1993) (Table 7.3). We also recommend the student to use the above systems only when an acetowhite area is observed.

Chapter 8

Colposcopic diagnosis of preclinical invasive carcinoma of the cervix and glandular neoplasia

- Acetowhite lesions with atypical vessels; large, complex acetowhite lesions obliterating the os; lesions with irregular and exophytic contour; strikingly thick, chalky-white lesions with raised and rolled out margins; and lesions bleeding on touch should be thoroughly investigated to rule out the possibility of early preclinical invasive cancer.

- Appearance of atypical blood vessels may indicate the first sign of invasion; one of the earliest colposcopic signs of invasion is blood vessels breaking out from mosaic formations.

- The atypical vessel patterns are varied and may take the form of hairpins, corkscrews, waste thread, commas, tadpole and other bizarre, irregular branching patterns with irregular calibre.

- Most glandular lesions originate in the transformation zone and may be associated with concomitant CIN lesions.

- Stark acetowhiteness of individual or fused villi in discrete patches in contrast to the surrounding columnar epithelium or closely placed, multiple cuffed crypt openings in a dense acetowhite lesion may indicate glandular lesions.

- Greyish-white, dense lesions with papillary excrescences and waste thread like or character writing-like atypical vessels or lesions with strikingly atypical villous structures may be associated with glandular lesions.

Invasive carcinoma is the stage of disease that follows CIN 3 or high-grade glandular intraepithelial neoplasia. Invasion implies that the neoplastic epithelial cells have invaded the stroma underlying the epithelium by breaching the basement membrane. The term preclinical invasive cancer is applied to very early invasive cancers (e.g., stage 1) in women without symptoms and gross physical findings and clinical signs, that are diagnosed incidentally during colposcopy or by other early-detection approaches such as screening. The primary responsibility of a colposcopist is to ensure that if preclinical invasive carcinoma of the cervix is present in a woman, it will be diagnosed. Colposcopic signs of this condition are usually recognizable early on, unless the lesion is hidden at the bottom of a crypt. This chapter describes the colposcopic detection of invasive

cervical carcinomas followed by a specific consideration of cervical glandular neoplasia.

It is crucial for the colposcopist to become familiar with the signs of preclinical cervical cancer and understand the need for strict adherence to the diagnostic protocols that ensure the safety of women who are referred into their care. The use of colposcopy and directed biopsy as a diagnostic approach replaces the use of cervical cold-knife conization as the main diagnostic approach to women with cervical abnormalities. This means that the onus for diagnostic accuracy no longer rests solely on the pathologist who evaluates the cone specimen, but also on the colposcopist who provides the histological material for the pathologist's examination. The use of ablative treatment such as cryotherapy, in which no histological specimen of the treated area is available, further highlights this responsibility for strict adherence to colposcopy protocol and familiarity with signs of invasive carcinoma.

Colposcopic approach

The colposcopist should be well aware that invasive cancers are more common in older women and in those referred with high-grade cytological abnormalities. Large high-grade lesions, involving more than three quadrants of the cervix, should be thoroughly investigated for the possibility of early invasive cancer, especially if associated with atypical vessels. Other warning signs include the presence of a wide abnormal transformation zone (greater than 40 mm^2), complex acetowhite lesions involving both lips of the cervix, lesions obliterating the os, lesions with irregular and exophytic surface contour, strikingly thick chalky white lesions with raised and rolled out margins, strikingly excessive atypical vessels, bleeding on touch or the presence of symptoms such as vaginal bleeding.

An advantage of performing a digital examination of the vagina and cervix before inserting the vaginal speculum is the opportunity to feel for any hint of nodularity or hardness of tissue. After the speculum is inserted, the cervix should have normal saline applied and the surface should be inspected for any suspicious lesions. Then the transformation zone should be identified, as described in Chapters 6 and 7.

Colposcopic examination proceeds in the normal fashion (Chapters 6 and 7) with successive applications of saline, acetic acid and Lugol's iodine solution and careful observation after each.

The colposcopic findings of preclinical invasive cervical cancer vary depending upon specific growth characteristics of the individual lesions, particularly early invasive lesions. The early preclinical invasive lesions turn densely greyish-white or yellowish-white very rapidly after the application of acetic acid (Figure 8.1). The acetowhiteness persists for several minutes.

One of the earliest colposcopic signs of possible invasion is blood vessels breaking out from the mosaic formations and producing irregular longitudinal vessels (Figure 8.2). As the neoplastic process closely approaches the stage of invasive cancer, the blood vessels can take on increasingly irregular, bizarre patterns. Appearance of atypical vessels usually indicates the first signs of invasion (Figures 8.1- 8.5). The key characteristics of these atypical surface vessels are that there is no gradual decrease in calibre (tapering) in the terminal branches and that the regular branching, seen in normal surface vessels, is absent. The atypical blood vessels, thought to be a result of horizontal pressure of the expanding neoplastic epithelium on the vascular spaces, show completely irregular and haphazard distribution, great variation in calibre with abrupt, angular changes in

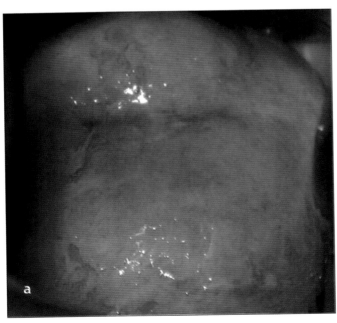 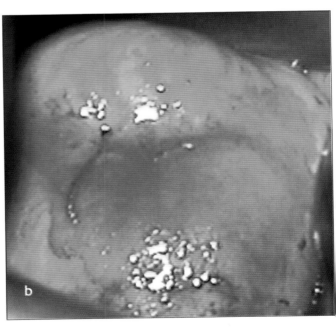

FIGURE 8.1: (a) There is a dense, opaque, thick acetowhite area involving all four quadrants of the cervix and extending into the endocervix, with irregular surface contour and atypical vessels

(b) The lesion is not taking up iodine and remains as a saffron yellow area after the application of Lugol's iodine solution

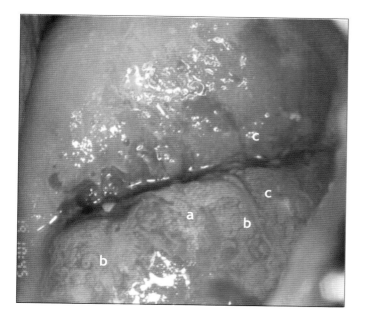

FIGURE 8.2: Early invasive cancer: Note the raised irregular mosaics with umbilication (a), breaking mosaics (b), surface irregularity and the atypical vessels (c) after the application of 5% acetic acid

direction with bizarre branching and patterns. These vessel shapes have been described by labels such as wide hairpin, waste thread, bizarre waste thread, cork screw, tendril, root-like or tree-like vessels (Figure 8.5).

They are irregular in size, shape, course and arrangement, and the intercapillary distance is substantially greater and more variable than that seen in normal epithelium.

If the cancer is predominantly exophytic, the lesion may appear as a raised growth with contact bleeding or capillary oozing. Early invasive carcinomas that are mainly exophytic tend to be soft and densely greyish-white in colour, with raised and rolled out margins (Figures 8.4 and 8.6). Surface bleeding or oozing is not uncommon, especially if there is a marked proliferation of atypical surface vessels (Figures 8.1-8.4 and 8.7). The bleeding may obliterate the acetowhiteness of the epithelium (Figures 8.2, 8.4 and 8.7). The atypical surface vessel types are varied and characteristically have widened intercapillary distances. These may take the form of hairpins, corkscrews, waste thread, commas, tadpole and other bizarre, irregular branching patterns and irregular calibre (Figures 8.1-8.5 and 8.7). The abnormal branching vessels show a pattern of large vessels suddenly becoming smaller and then abruptly opening up again into a larger vessel. All of these abnormalities can best be detected with the green (or blue) filter and the use of a higher power of magnification. Proper

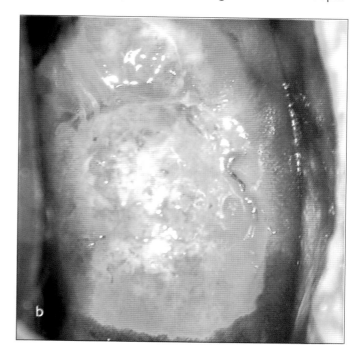

FIGURE 8.3: Early invasive cancer: (a) There is a large, dense, opaque acetowhite area with an irregular surface contour, coarse punctations and atypical vessels, involving all four quadrants of the cervix. There are internal borders within the acetowhite areas (arrows). The are several cuffed crypt openings
(b) The lesion does not take up iodine and remains as a mustard yellow area after the application of Lugol's iodine

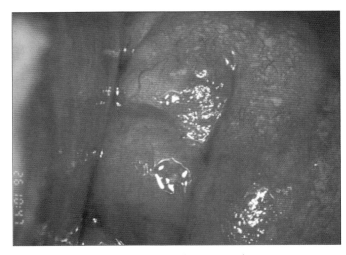

Appearance before application of acetic acid

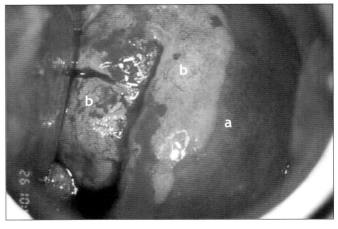

Appearance after application of 5% acetic acid

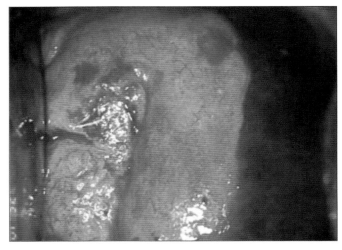

Appearance after application of Lugol's iodine

FIGURE 8.4: Early invasive cancer: Note the thick, dense, opaque acetowhite lesions with raised and rolled out margins (a) and atypical vessels (b) which started to bleed after touch. Note the mustard-yellow iodine-negative area corresponding to the extent of the lesion. Irregular surface with "mountains-and-valleys" pattern is evident

evaluation of these abnormal vessel patterns, particularly with the green filter, constitutes a very important step in the colposcopic diagnosis of early invasive cervical cancers.

Early preclinical invasive cancer may also appear as dense, thick, chalky-white areas with surface irregularity and nodularity and with raised and rolled out margins (Figure 8.6). Such lesions may not present atypical blood vessel patterns and may not bleed on touch. Irregular surface contour with a mountains- and valleys- appearance is also characteristic of early invasive cancers (Figures 8.2-8.4, 8.6 and 8.7). Colposcopically suspect early, preclinical invasive cancers are often very extensive, complex lesions involving all the quadrants of the cervix. Such lesions frequently involve the endocervical canal and may obliterate the external os. Infiltrating lesions appear as hard nodular white areas and may present necrotic areas in the centre. Invasive cancers of the cervix rarely produce glycogen and therefore, the lesions turn mustard yellow or saffron yellow after application of Lugol's iodine (Figures 8.1, 8.3, 8.4 and 8.7).

If a biopsy is taken of a lesion that is suspicious for invasive carcinoma and the report is negative for invasion, the responsibility rests with the colposcopist to ensure that a possibly more generous biopsy and an endocervical curettage (ECC) be taken at a subsequent examination. It is mandatory to take another biopsy if the pathologist reports that there is inadequate stromal tissue present on which to base a pathological decision as to whether invasion is present.

Advanced, frankly invasive cancers do not necessarily require colposcopy for diagnosis (Figures 3.4-3.6 and 8.8). A properly conducted vaginal speculum examination with digital palpation should establish the diagnosis so that further confirmatory and staging investigations may be performed. Biopsy should be taken from the periphery of the growth, avoiding areas of necrosis, to ensure accurate histopathological diagnosis.

Glandular lesions:

There are no obvious colposcopic features that allow definite diagnosis of adenocarcinoma *in situ* (AIS) and adenocarcinoma, as no firm criteria have been established and widely accepted for recognizing glandular lesions. Most cervical AIS or early adenocarcinoma is discovered incidentally after biopsy for squamous intraepithelial neoplasia. It is worth noting that often AIS coexists with CIN. The colposcopic

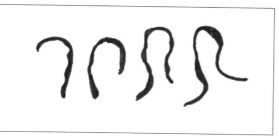

(a): Wide hair pin-like vessels

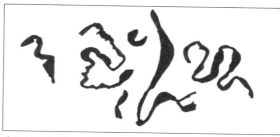

(b): Waste thread vessels

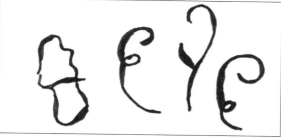

(c): Tendril-like vessels

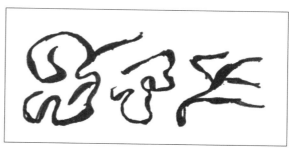

(d): Bizarre branching waste thread vessels

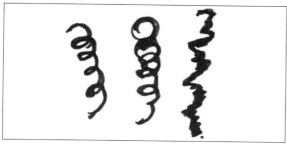

(e): Corkscrew vessels

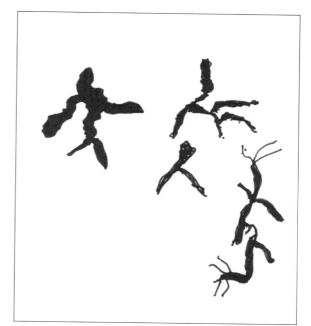

(f): Irregular root-like vessels

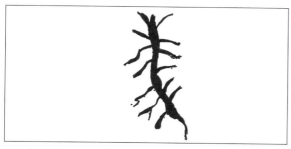

(g): Tree-like vessels

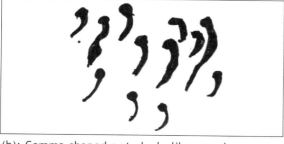

(h): Comma-shaped or tadpole-like vessels

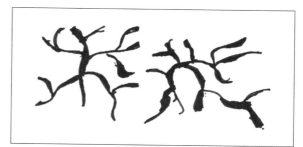

(i): Irregular branching vessels

FIGURE 8.5: Atypical vessel patterns

diagnosis of AIS and adenocarcinoma require a high degree of training and skill.

It has been suggested that most glandular lesions originate within the transformation zone and colposcopic recognition of the stark acetowhiteness of either the individual or fused villi in discrete patches (in contrast to the surrounding pinkish white columnar villi) may lead to a colposcopic suspicion of glandular lesions. While CIN lesions are almost always

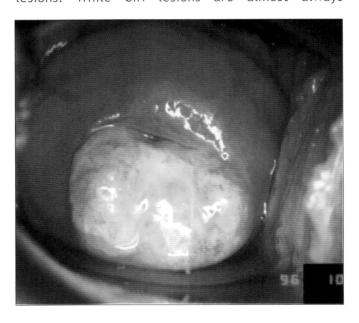

FIGURE 8.6: Dense, chalky white complex acetowhite lesion with raised and rolled out margin and irregular, nodular surface suggestive of early invasive cancer

connected with the squamocolumnar junction, glandular lesions may present densely white island lesions in the columnar epithelium (Figure 8.9). In approximately half of women with AIS, the lesion is entirely within the canal (Figure 8.9) and may easily be missed if the endocervical canal is not properly visualized and investigated.

A lesion in the columnar epithelium containing branch-like or root-like vessels (Figure 8.5) may also suggest glandular disease. Strikingly acetowhite columnar villi in stark contrast to the surrounding villi may suggest glandular lesions (Figure 8.10). Elevated lesions with an irregular acetowhite surface, papillary patterns and atypical blood vessels overlying the columnar epithelium may be associated with glandular lesions (Figure 8.11). A variegated patchy red and white lesion with small papillary excrescences and epithelial buddings and large crypt openings in the columnar epithelium may also be associated with glandular lesions.

Invasive adenocarcinoma may present as greyish-white dense acetowhite lesions with papillary excrescences and waste thread-like or character writing-like atypical blood vessels (Figure 8.12). The soft surface may come off easily when touched with a cotton applicator. Adenocarcinoma may also present as strikingly atypical villous structures with atypical vessels replacing normal ectocervical columnar epithelium (Figure 8.13). Closely placed, multiple cuffed crypt openings in a dense acetowhite lesion

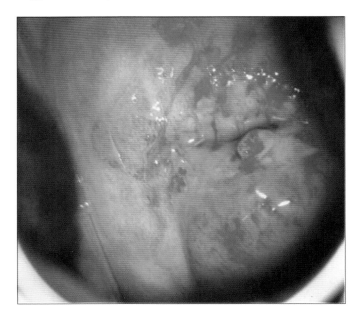

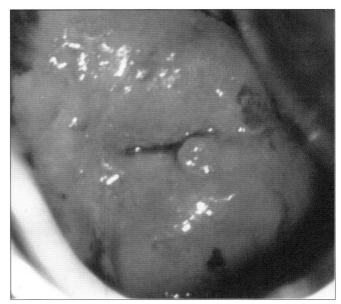

FIGURE 8.7: Invasive cervical cancer: (a) note the irregular surface contour with mountains-and-valleys appearance with atypical blood vessels in the dense acetowhite area; (b) appearance after the application of Lugol's iodine

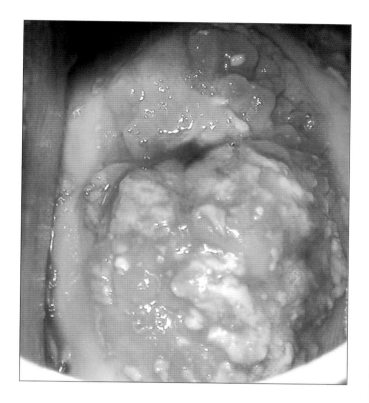

FIGURE 8.8: Invasive cancer: There is a proliferative growth on the cervix which becomes dense, chalky white after the application of acetic acid. Bleeding partly obliterates the acetowhitening

with irregular surface may also indicate a glandular lesion (Figure 8.14).

In summary, the accurate colposcopic diagnosis of preclinical invasive carcinoma and glandular lesions depends on several factors: continuing alertness on the part of the colposcopist, strict adherence to the step-by-step approach to examination, the use of a grading index, close attention to surface blood vessels, the honest appraisal of when an examination is inadequate, the appropriate use of ECC to rule out lesions in the canal, and the taking of a well directed biopsy of sufficient tissue on which to base a reliable histopathological diagnosis.

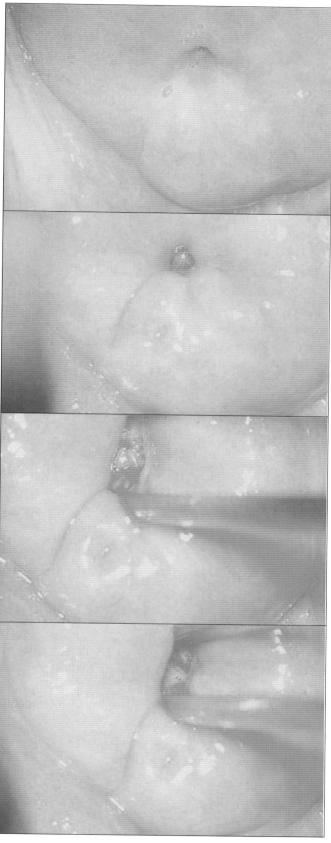

FIGURE 8.9: A dense acetowhite lesion in the endocervical canal visible after stretching the os with a long dissection forceps (adenocarcinoma *in situ*).

75

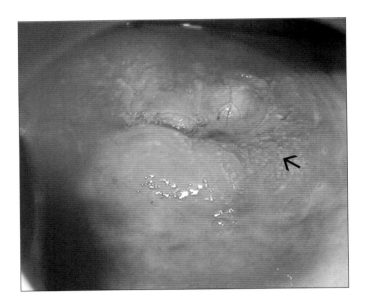

FIGURE 8.10: Adenocarcinoma *in situ* : The tips of some of the columnar villi turn densely white compared to the surrounding columnar villi after the application of acetic acid (arrow). The nabothian cysts turn white after the application of acetic acid

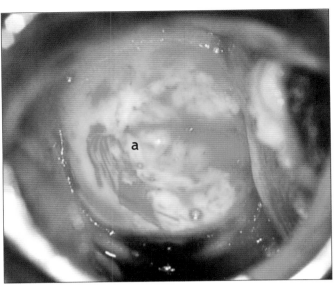

FIGURE 8.12: Adenocarcinoma: Note the greyish-white dense acetowhite lesion with character writing-like atypical blood vessels (a)

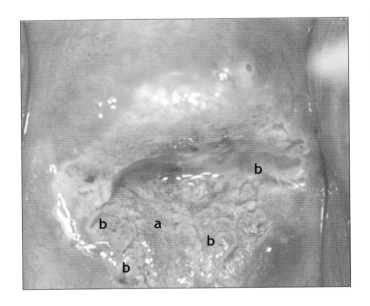

FIGURE 8.11: Adenocarcinoma *in situ*: Note the elevated lesions with an irregular acetowhite surface, enlarged and hypertrophied villi, papillary patterns (a), and atypical vessels (b), overlying the columnar epithelium

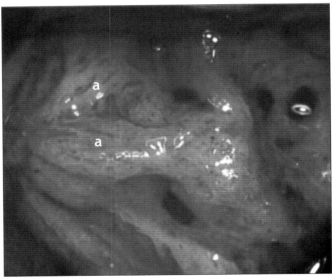

FIGURE 8.13: Adenocarcinoma: Note the elongated, dense acetowhite lesion with irregular surface in the columnar epithelium with atypical blood vessels (a)

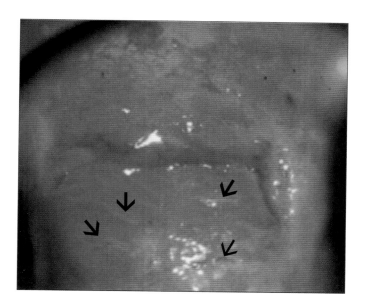

FIGURE 8.14: Adenocarcinoma: Note the multiple cuffed crypt openings (narrow arrow) in a dense acetowhite lesion with irregular surface and the hypertrophied columnar villi (dense arrows) in the columnar epithelium

Inflammatory lesions of the uterine cervix

- The inflammatory lesions of cervical and vaginal mucosa are associated with excessive, malodorous or non-odourous, frothy or non-frothy, grey or greenish-yellow or white discharge and symptoms such as lower abdominal pain, back ache, pruritus, itching, and dyspareunia.

- Colposcopic features of cervical inflammation such as inflammatory punctation, congestion and ulceration as well as ill-defined, patchy acetowhitening are widely and diffusely distributed in the cervix and vagina and not restricted to the transformation zone.

Inflammatory lesions of the cervix and vagina are commonly observed, and particularly in women living in tropical developing countries. Cervical inflammation is mostly due to infection (usually mixed or polymicrobial); other causes include foreign bodies (an intrauterine device, a retained tampon, etc.), trauma, and chemical irritants such as gels or creams. The clinical features and diagnostic characteristics of these lesions are described in this chapter to help in the differential diagnosis of cervical lesions.

The inflammatory lesions are associated with mucopurulent, seropurulent, white or serous discharge and symptoms such as lower abdominal pain, backache, pruritus, itching and dyspareunia. As stated earlier, they are most commonly caused by infections or irritating foreign bodies. Common infectious organisms responsible for such lesions include protozoan infections with *Trichomonas vaginalis*; fungal infections such as *Candida albicans*; overgrowth of anaerobic bacteria (Bacteroides, Peptostreptococcus, *Gardnerella vaginalis*, *Gardnerella mobiluncus*) in a condition such as bacterial vaginosis; other bacteria such as *Chlamydia trachomatis*, *Haemophilus ducreyi*, *Mycoplasma hominis*, Streptococcus, *Escherichia coli*, Staphylococcus, and *Neisseria gonorrhoea*; and infections with viruses such as herpes simplex virus.

Women with cervical inflammation suffer every day with pruritic or non-pruritic, purulent or non-purulent, malodorous or non-odorous discharge, frothy or non-frothy discharge, which stain their underclothes, necessitating regular use of sanitary pads. These inflammatory conditions are thus symptomatic and should be identified, differentiated from cervical neoplasia, and treated. A biopsy should be taken whenever in doubt.

Examination of the external anogenitalia, vagina and cervix for vesicles, shallow ulcers and button-like ulcers and the inguinal region for inflamed and/or enlarged lymph nodes, and lower abdominal and bimanual palpation for pelvic tenderness and mass should be part of the clinical examination to rule out infective conditions.

Cervicovaginitis

The term *cervicovaginitis* refers to inflammation of the squamous epithelium of the vagina and cervix. In cervicovaginitis, the cervical and vaginal mucosa respond to infection with an inflammatory reaction that is characterized by damage to surface cells. This damage leads to desquamation and ulceration, which cause a reduction in the epithelial thickness due to loss of superficial and part of the intermediate layers of cells (which contain glycogen). In the deeper layers, the cells are swollen with infiltration of neutrophils in the intercellular space. The surface of the epithelium is covered by cellular debris and inflammatory mucopurulent secretions. The underlying connective tissue is congested with dilatation of the superficial vessels and with enlarged and dilated stromal papillae.

Cervicitis

Cervicitis is the term used to denote the inflammation

involving the columnar epithelium of the cervix. It results in congestion of underlying connective tissue, desquamation of cells and ulceration with mucopurulent discharge. If the inflammation persists, the villous structures become flattened, and the grape-like appearance is lost and the mucosa may secrete less mucus.

In both the above conditions, after repeated inflammation and tissue necrosis, the lesions are repaired and necrotic tissue is eliminated. The newly formed epithelium has numerous vessels, and connective tissue proliferation results in fibrosis of varying extent.

Colposcopic appearances
Before the application of acetic acid

Examination, before application of acetic acid, reveals moderate to excessive cervical and vaginal secretions, which may sometimes indicate the nature of underlying infection. In *T. vaginalis* infection (trichomoniasis), which is very common in tropical areas, there is copious, bubbly, frothy, malodorous, greenish-yellow, mucopurulent discharge. Bacterial infections are associated with thin, liquid, seropurulent discharge. The secretion may be foul-smelling in the case of anaerobic bacterial overgrowth, bacterial vaginosis, and *Trichomonas* infection. In the case of candidiasis (moniliasis) and other yeast infections, the secretion is thick and curdy (cheesy) white with intense itching resulting in a reddened vulva. Foul-smelling, dark-coloured mucopurulent discharges are associated with inflammatory states due to foreign bodies (e.g., a retained tampon). Gonorrhoea results in purulent vaginal discharge and cervical tenderness. Small vesicles filled with serous fluid may be observed in the cervix and vagina in the vesicular phase of herpes simplex viral infection. Herpetic infections are associated with episodes of painful vulvar, vaginal and cervical ulceration lasting for two weeks. Excoriation marks are evident with trichomoniasis, moniliasis and mixed bacterial infections.

A large coalesced ulcer due to herpes, or other inflammatory conditions, may mimic the appearance of invasive cancer. Chronic inflammation may cause recurrent ulceration and healing of the cervix, resulting in distortion of the cervix due to healing by fibrosis. There may be associated necrotic areas as well. A biopsy should be directed if in doubt. Rare and uncommon cervical infections, due to tuberculosis,

schistosomiasis and amoebiasis, cause extensive ulceration and necrosis of the cervix with symptoms and signs mimicking invasive cancer; a biopsy will confirm the diagnosis.

If the infectious process is accompanied by marked ulceration (with or without necrosis), the ulcerated area may be covered with purulent exudate, with marked differences in the surface level of the cervix. There may be exudation of serous droplets.

Longstanding bacterial, fungal or protozoal infection and inflammation may lead to fibrosis, which appears white or pink, depending on the degree of fibrosis. The epithelium covering the connective tissue is fragile, leading to ulceration and bleeding. Appearances following acetic acid and iodine application are variable, depending on the integrity of the surface epithelium.

In the case of cervicitis, the columnar epithelium is intensely red, bleeds on contact and opaque purulent discharge is present. The columnar villous or grape-like appearance may be lost due to flattening of the villi, to repeated inflammation and to the fact that there are no clearly defined papillae (Figure 9.1). Extensive areas of the cervix and infected vaginal mucosa appear red due to congestion of the underlying connective tissue.

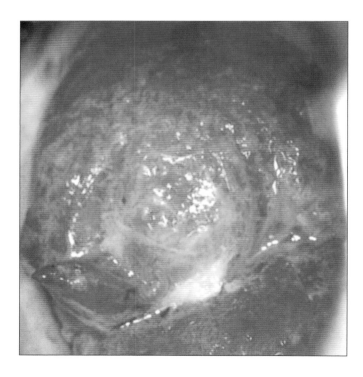

FIGURE 9.1: Reddish "angry-looking", inflamed columnar epithelium with loss of the villous structure and with inflammatory exudate (before application of 5% acetic acid)

After application of acetic acid

The liberal application of acetic acid clears the cervix and vagina of secretions, but may cause pain. Cervicovaginitis is associated with oedema, capillary dilatation, enlargement of the stromal papillae, which contain the vascular bundles, and infiltration of the

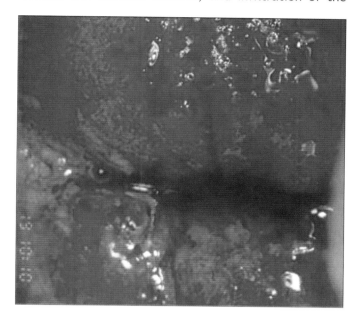

FIGURE 9.2: Chronic cervicitis: this cervix is extensively inflamed with a reddish appearance and bleeding on touch; there are ill-defined, patchy acetowhite areas scattered all over the cervix after the application of acetic acid

stroma with inflammatory cells. Chronically inflamed cervix may appear reddish, with ill-defined, patchy acetowhite areas scattered in the cervix, not restricted to the transformation zone and may bleed on touch (Figures 9.2, 9.3). The enlarged stromal papillae appear as red spots (red punctation) in a pinkish-white background, usually in the case of *T. vaginalis* infection, after application of acetic acid. An inexperienced colposcopist may confuse the inflammatory punctations with those seen in cervical intraepithelial neoplasia (CIN). However, one can differentiate using the following criteria: inflammatory punctations are fine, with extremely minimal intercapillary distances, and diffusely distributed (not restricted to the transformation zone) and they involve the original squamous epithelium and vagina with intervening inflamed mucosa. As the inflammation persists and becomes chronic, it results in large, focal red punctations due to large collections of capillaries grouped together, which appear as several red spots of different sizes visible in a pinkish-white background, producing the so-called 'strawberry spots' (Figure 9.4). Colposcopically, a chronically inflamed cervix may sometimes resemble invasive cervical cancer (Figure 9.5).

After application of Lugol's iodine

The test outcome after application of Lugol's iodine solution depends upon the desquamation and the loss

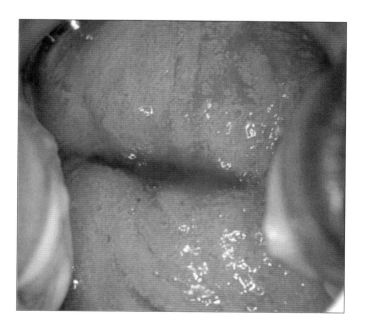

FIGURE 9.3: Chronic cervicitis: the cervix is highly inflamed and eroded with ill-defined, patchy acetowhite areas scattered all over

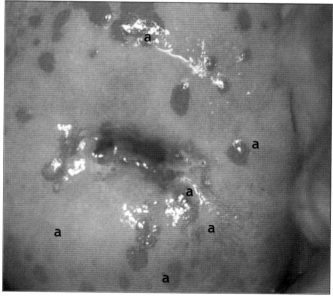

FIGURE 9.4: Multiple red spots (a) suggestive of *Trichomonas vaginalis* colpitis (strawberry appearance) (after application of 5% acetic acid)

81

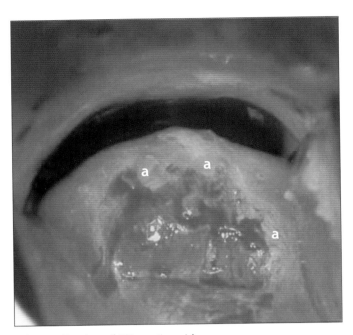

After application of 5% acetic acid

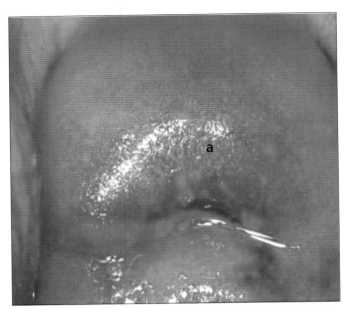

FIGURE 9.6: Stippled appearance (a) due to *Trichomonas vaginalis* colpitis after application of Lugol's iodine

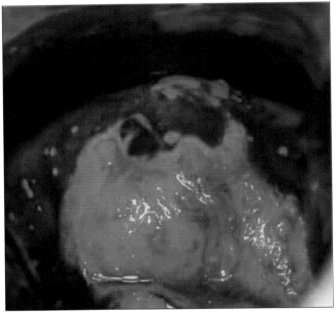

After application of Lugol's iodine

FIGURE 9.5: Colposcopic appearance of a chronically inflamed cervix showing areas of ulceration, necrosis and healing. The regenerating areas turn somewhat white (a) after application of acetic acid. The inflamed areas do not take up iodine

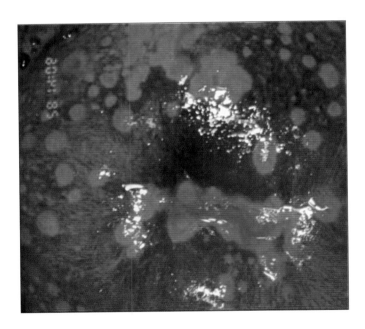

FIGURE 9.7: *Trichomonas vaginalis* colpitis after application of Lugol's iodine (leopard-skin appearance)

of cell layers containing glycogen. If desquamation is limited to the summit of the stromal papillae where the squamous epithelium is thinnest, a series of thin yellow spots are seen on a mahogany-brown background, giving a stippled appearance (Figure 9.6). When the inflammation persists and the infection becomes chronic, the small desquamated areas become confluent to form large desquamated areas leading to the so-called leopard-skin appearance (Figure 9.7). These features are often found with *Trichomonas* infection, but also may be seen with fungal and bacterial infections. If there is marked desquamation, the cervix appears yellowish-red in colour, with involvement of vagina (Figure 9.8).

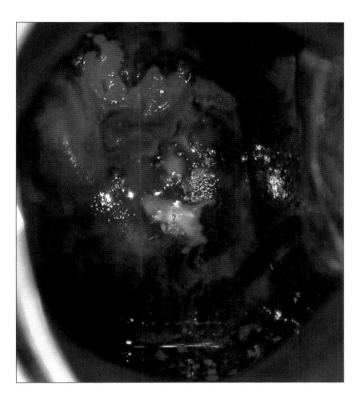

FIGURE 9.8: Chronic cervicitis: there are scattered, ill-defined, patchy iodine non-uptake areas on the cervix and vagina. Also, the cervix appears yellowish red in colour

In summary, inflammatory conditions of the cervix are associated with excessive, usually malodorous, mucopurulent, seropurulent or whitish discharge, red punctations, ulceration, and healing by fibrosis. The secretion is frothy with bubbles in the case of trichomoniasis and sticky cheese white in candidiasis. Inflammatory lesions of the cervix may be differentiated from CIN by their large, diffuse involvement of the cervix, extension to the vagina, red colour tone and associated symptoms such as discharge and pruritus.

Avoiding errors in the colposcopic assessment of the cervix and colposcopic provisional diagnosis

- A thorough knowledge of anatomy, pathophysiology and natural history of diseases of the female genital tract is essential to avoid errors in colposcopic assessment.

- Strict adherence to a diagnostic protocol and an awareness of the limitations of colposcopy are equally important.

- Regular interaction with the pathologists and clinical audits help to improve the quality of colposcopy.

- We encourage arriving at a provisional diagnosis, based on the colposcopic findings.

An adequate knowledge of pathophysiology and understanding of the natural history of diseases of the female genital tract that can be diagnosed with the colposcope and then treated are essential for satisfactory performance of colposcopy. A thorough knowledge of instrumentation, methods of examination and terminology is equally important. A high degree of accuracy in diagnosing cervical intraepithelial neoplasia (CIN) and ruling out invasive cancer may be achieved with good clinical judgement. Scrupulous adherence to a diagnostic protocol and awareness of the limitations and pitfalls of colposcopy are important.

Errors are commonly committed due to a lack of awareness and to deviation from established colposcopic protocol and practice. Good training, experience, an innate interest, and an established diagnostic algorithm will diminish the possibility of errors. These factors are particularly important in low-resource environments, where there are limited opportunities for mutual consultations and continuing education. The colposcopist should try to achieve the same degree of accuracy as a histopathologist can achieve with cervical conization specimens.

A summary of common sources of shortcomings in colposcopic practice is presented in Table 10.1. Regular interaction with the pathologist and clinical audits, to correlate colposcopic diagnoses with histological diagnoses, helps to improve the quality of colposcopy. It is important for the provider to learn the art of taking colposcopically directed biopsies from appropriate area(s) in the transformation zone by using sharp biopsy forceps without crushing specimens. If the squamocolumnar junction is hidden in the endocervical canal, it is necessary to perform endocervical curettage (ECC) or cone biopsy in order to investigate the canal properly. It is obligatory to wait for 60 seconds after a liberal application of acetic acid for it to take full effect. Specific mention should be made of the location of the squamocolumnar junction and the acetowhite areas in relation to the junction. Careful inspection of the vagina should also be made for any extension of cervical lesions. It is best to examine the vagina when the speculum is being withdrawn at the end of each examination. Findings must be clearly and legibly documented. Using an objective scoring system such as Reid's score (Appendix 5) is particularly helpful for beginners to arrive at a colposcopic diagnosis and to select appropriate sites for directed biopsies. Continuing education is important to enable the colposcopist to keep up with developments. Avoidance of missing or undertreating an invasive cancer and ensuring the provision of adequate treatment is largely dependent on the skills of the colposcopist.

Colposcopic provisional diagnosis
We strongly encourage the colposcopists to make a provisional diagnosis, based on the findings of

Table 10.1: Common sources of colposcopic errors

Inadequate training and experience

Inadequate understanding of the natural history of disease

Failure to use an established diagnostic protocol or deviation from the protocol

Failure to use the largest speculum possible

False squamocolumnar junction caused by abrasion

Failure to choose appropriate biopsy sites and failure to take enough biopsies

Failure to take a biopsy when in doubt

Using a blunt, non-sharp biopsy punch to obtain tissue specimens

Failure to take a colposcopically directed biopsy

Failure to perform biopsies from condylomata or leukoplakia

Failure to wait for the full effect of acetic acid

Failure to apply Lugol's iodine solution and examine

Failure to examine the endocervical canal adequately when the lesion limit or squamocolumnar junction is not seen

Failure to do endocervical curettage (ECC) when the lesion limit is not seen

Failure to perform excision when the lesion limit is not seen with an endocervical speculum or when ECC is equivocal or positive

Failure to perform excision when microinvasion is suspected

Failure to inspect the vagina and vulva

Failure to properly and legibly record colposcopic findings

Failure to communicate with the pathologist

Failure to correlate histological and colposcopic findings

Failure to consult experts in difficult cases

Failure to keep up with continuing education

Failure to self-audit

Adapted from: Popkin (1995)

colposcopic examination. The provisional diagnosis may be in terms of normal, inflammation, leukoplakia, condyloma, low-grade CIN, high-grade CIN, early invasive cancer, overt invasive cancer, others (atrophy, cervical polyp, radiation changes, etc.) and inconclusive. Such diagnosis is based on the evaluation of all the findings such as the characteristics of the acetowhite areas, vascular features, colour change after iodine application, surface characteristics such as ulceration, and other signs such as bleeding on touch, the nature of cervical and vaginal discharge and the findings of examination of external anogenitalia, groin and lower abdomen. These are described in detail in Chapters 6-9. Once a provisional diagnosis is made, a plan for management of the condition diagnosed should be developed. Table 10.2 provides a summary of the colposcopic findings that help in making the provisional diagnosis.

Table 10.2: A summary of colposcopic features guiding provisional diagnosis

Diagnosis	Colour tone	Acetowhitening		Relation to TZ and SCJ	Duration of effect	Vascular features	Iodine uptake	Bleeding on touch	Ulceration	Discharge
		Demarcation	Margin	Surface						
Normal	-	-	-	-	-	-	Normal vascular pattern	Squamous epithelium black in colour; columnar epithelium, no change in colour	Nil	Nil	Clear secretion from the columnar epithelium
Normal, immature metaplasia	Pinkish white, or snow white, translucent, patchy acetowhite areas	Nil	Indistinct, blends with the rest of the epithelium	Smooth; crypt openings, islands of columnar epithelium seen	Restricted to TZ; prominent near the SCJ	< 1 minute	Normal vascular pattern	No or partial uptake	Nil	Nil	Clear secretion from the columnar epithelium
Normal, mature metaplasia	Light pinkish white hue. No confluent acetowhite area	Nil	Blends with the rest of the epithelium	Smooth, reveals crypt openings, nabothian follicles	Restricted to TZ	-	Normal vascular pattern	Takes up iodine, turns black or brown	Nil	Nil	Clear secretion from the columnar epithelium
Inflammation	Pale, patchy areas, with intervening red areas and/or necrotic areas	Nil	Indistinct, blends with the rest of the epithelium	Irregular, variegated appearance	Not restricted to TZ, may be widely disseminated	< 2 minutes	Diffusely distributed, fine red punctation involving cervix and vagina	Partial iodine uptake	May be present	May be present	Malodorous, profuse, mucopurulent or seropurulent or non-odorous thick, sticky, white discharge
Low-grade CIN	Moderately dense, shiny, opaque, thin lesions	Well demarcated confluent lesions	Irregular, feathery, jagged, digitating, angular or geographic	Flat, smooth or microcondyloma-tous or micropapillary	Mostly seen in the TZ, abuts the SCJ. Very early lesions may be outside TZ as satellite lesions	1-2 minutes	Fine punctation and/or mosaic with in the AW lesion may be seen	No uptake	Nil	Nil	Nil

Table 10.2 (cont.): A summary of colposcopic features guiding provisional diagnosis

| Diagnosis | Acetowhitening | | | | | | | | | |
	Colour tone	Demarcation	Margin	Surface	Relation to TZ and SCJ	Duration of effect	Vascular features	Iodine uptake	Bleeding on touch	Ulceration	Discharge
High-grade CIN	Dull, dense, greyish-white or oyster-white opaque lesion	Well demarcated confluent lesions; internal demarcations and borders may be present	Regular, smooth outlines; occasionally may be raised and rolled out	Less smooth, more irregular and/or occasionally nodular surface	Restricted to TZ, abutting the SCJ	2-4 minutes	Coarse punctation and/or coarse mosaic within the AW lesion may be seen; atypical vessels may be seen (+)	No iodine uptake	May be present in severe lesions	Nil	Nil
Preclinical invasive cancer	Chalky white, thick, dense, opaque lesions	Well demarcated	Raised and rolled out margins	Irregular, nodular or mountains- and-valley pattern	May involve the entire cervix, large complex lesions obliterating the os	> 3 minutes	Coarse raised mosaics and/or breaking mosaics and/or, coarse punctations; atypical vessels always present (+++++)	No iodine uptake	Surface bleeding/-oozing common	May be seen	May be present due to secondary infection
Overt invasive cancer	Dense white areas, may be obliterated by profuse bleeding	Entire cervix replaced by growth	Entire cervix replaced by growth	Ulceropro-liferative growth	Entire cervix replaced by growth extending to adjacent tissues	Whiteness usually obliterated by bleeding	Atypical vessels always present (++++++)	No uptake, but bleeding obliterates iodine uptake patterns	Profuse bleeding	Always present	Malodorous, blood stained, purulent discharge due to secondary infection

TZ: transformation zone ; SCJ: squamocolumnar junction; AW: Acetowhitening

Chapter 11

Management that provides continuity of care for women

- If women are diagnosed with reproductive tract infection, prompt treatment should be instituted according to the WHO guidelines.

- Though it may be preferred to have the diagnosis of CIN firmly established before treatment is offered, in many low-resource settings, treatment may be offered at the first colposcopy visit, based on colposcopic findings, to maximize treatment coverage.

- The clinical management of women with CIN 1 lesions may take one of the following courses: (i) immediate treatment or (ii) follow the woman and then treat if the lesion is persistent or progressive after 18 to 24 months.

- All women with CIN 2 and CIN 3 lesions should be treated with cryotherapy or LEEP.

- Women diagnosed with invasive cancer should be promptly referred for treatment.

- Women diagnosed with high-grade CIN during pregnancy can be reviewed at about 28 weeks gestation. If the disease is stable, the woman may be reviewed at 2-3 months post-partum for definitive diagnosis by biopsy and appropriate management of lesions.

- Women treated for CIN may be reviewed at 9-12 months after treatment.

Planning a woman's medical management after her initial colposcopic assessment is primarily the duty of the colposcopist. It is appropriate to involve the woman, as a partner, in the decision-making process. Management usually depends on the final assessment after the colposcopic findings have been integrated with the pathology reports. Management plans also depend on whether or not the woman is pregnant. The management plan should be explicitly detailed in the medical record and communicated clearly to the patient at the earliest opportunity. Ideally, pathology reports (biopsy, endocervical curettage (ECC), loop electrosurgical excision procedure (LEEP) specimen, cytology) should be available to the colposcopist within three weeks of carrying out the colposcopy. Cryotherapy or LEEP are the two forms of therapy discussed in this manual (see Chapters 12 and 13), but it must be emphasized each has specific indications for

their use and should be used only when women fulfil all of the eligibility criteria for the specific therapy. A general plan of management that may be adapted in low-resource settings is shown in Figure 11.1.

It is generally preferable to have the diagnosis of cervical intraepithelial neoplasia (CIN) firmly established before a decision on management is taken and any treatment offered. However, there may be exceptions to this rule. For example, in many settings, particularly developing countries, women may be offered treatment at their first colposcopy visit, based on colposcopic assessment to maximize treatment coverage (otherwise patients lost to follow-up would not receive treatment for lesions). If the decision is to treat with cryotherapy, a biopsy (or biopsies) may be directed before cryotherapy, as this type of treatment does not produce a tissue specimen for histological examination. A tissue sample taken before instituting

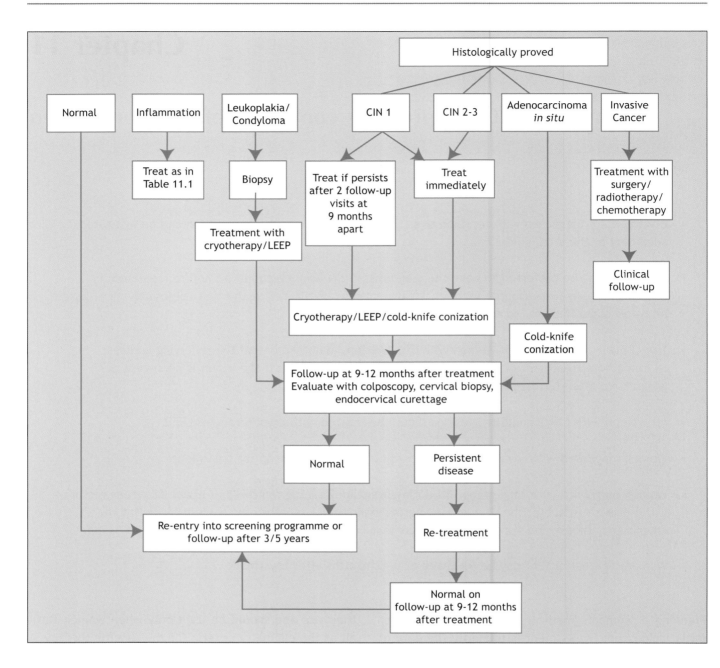

FIGURE 11.1: Flow chart of management decisions in cervical neoplasia and other conditions in low-resource settings. (CIN-cervical intraepithelial neoplasia; LEEP-Loop electrosurgical excision procedure)

ablative therapy will help to confirm the histological nature of the lesion treated a *posteriori*. Expert colposcopists also may use this approach to maximize treatment coverage and to minimize the number of clinic visits in some settings. However, this approach may result in a significant degree of overtreatment. Even though it is assumed that treatment methods such cryotherapy and LEEP are safe, and are unlikely to be associated with long-term sequelae and complications, the long-term implications of such overtreatment remains yet to be firmly established. On the other hand, it is likely that overtreatment may, to a certain

extent, protect against future development of CIN, in view of the ablation of the transformation zone where the vast majority of CIN lesions occur.

Outcomes after colposcopic assessment
Normal colposcopy outcome

In most women with a normal cervix, assessment using the colposcope results in a satisfactory evaluation of the cervix. If the squamocolumnar junction is visible and there is no colposcopic evidence of CIN or invasive cancer, the woman should be discharged and may resume participation in the screening programme, if one is on-going in the region (which is not the case in many developing countries!). Otherwise, she may be advised to undergo a repeat screening examination after three to five years.

Reproductive tract infection

If a woman is diagnosed with reproductive tract infection, prompt treatment should be instituted following the WHO guidelines (WHO, 2001). The

Table 11.1 Treatment for reproductive tract infections

Reproductive tract infection	Treatment guidelines	
	Non-pregnant women	Pregnant women
T. vaginalis (Trichomoniasis)	Metronidazole 400 mg orally, 2 times a day, for 7 days or tinidazole 500 mg orally, 2 times a day, for 7 days or a single dose of metronidazole 2 g orally or tinidazole 2 g orally.	1st trimester: Metronidazole gel, 0.75%, 5 g, 2 times a day intravaginally, for 7 days; 2nd and 3rd trimester: same as non-pregnant women.
Candidiasis	Clotrimazole or miconazole, 200 mg intravaginally, daily for 3 days or Fluconazole, 150 mg orally, as a single dose.	Clotrimazole or miconazole, 200 mg intravaginally, daily for 3 days.
Bacterial vaginosis	Metronidazole 400 mg orally, 2 times a day, for 7 days.	Metronidazole gel, 0.75%, 5 g, 2 times a day intravaginally, for 7 days or clindamycin, 300 mg orally, 2 times daily, for 7 days.
Chlamydial infection	Doxycycline 100 mg orally, 2 times a day, for 7 days or azithromycin, 1 g orally, as a single dose.	Erythromycin 500 mg orally, 4 times daily, for 7 days or amoxycillin, 500 mg orally, 3 times daily, for 7 days.
Gonococcal infection	Ciprofloxacin, 500 mg, orally, as a single dose or azithromycin 2 g orally as a single dose.	Cefixime, 200 mg orally, as a single dose or ceftriaxone, 125 mg intramuscularly, as a single dose.
Syphilis	Benzathine penicillin, 2.4 million IU, by intramuscular injection, as a single treatment; in penicillin-allergic patients, doxycycline, 100 mg orally, 2 times a day, for 15 days	Benzathine penicillin, 2.4 million IU, by intramuscular injection, as a single treatment; in penicillin-allergic patients, erythromycin 500 mg orally, 4 times daily, for 15 days.
Lymphogranuloma venereum	Doxycycline, 100 mg orally, 2 times daily, for 14 days or erythromycin 500 mg orally, 4 times a day, for 14 days.	Erythromycin 500 mg orally, 4 times a day, for 14 days.
Chancroid	Ciprofloxacin, 500 mg orally, 2 times a day, for 3 days or erythromycin 500 mg orally, 4 times a day, for 7 days or a single dose of azithromycin, 1 g orally.	Erythromycin 500 mg orally, 4 times a day, for 7 days.
Granuloma inguinale	Azithromycin, 1 g orally, as a single dose or doxycycline, 100 mg orally, 2 times daily, for 14 days	Erythromycin 500 mg orally, 4 times a day, for 7 days.
Genital herpes	Acyclovir, 400 mg orally, 3 times daily, for 7 days or famciclovir, 250 mg orally, 3 times daily, for 7 days.	-
Pelvic inflammatory disease (PID)	Ceftriaxone 250 mg as a single intramuscular injection plus doxycycline 100 mg orally, 2 times a day, for 14 days or cefixime 800 mg orally as a single dose plus doxycycline as above or Ciprofloxacin 500 mg orally as a single dose plus doxycycline as above.	Erythromycin 500 mg orally, 4 times a day, for 14 days.

treatment policies for pregnant and non-pregnant women, diagnosed with reproductive tract infection, are outlined in Table 11.1. Use of oral metronidazole is contraindicated during the first trimester of pregnancy, but can be safely used in the second and third trimesters. Patients taking oral metronidazole should be cautioned not to consume alcohol while they are taking the drug or up to 24 hours after taking the last dose. Patients with advanced syphilis may require prolonged treatment with antibiotics. There is no known cure for genital herpes infections, but the course of symptoms can be modified if systemic therapy with acyclovir or its analogues is initiated.

Leukoplakia (hyperkeratosis)

Leukoplakia should be biopsied and submitted for histopathological examination, to rule out underlying cervical neoplasia.

Condyloma

Condylomata should be biopsied and localized ectocervical exophytic lesions may be treated with ablative treatment by cryotherapy or electrofulguration or with excisional treatment such as LEEP.

CIN 1

If the final diagnosis in a woman is CIN 1, the clinical management may take one of the following courses: either to (a) to immediately treat the lesion or (b) follow the woman cytologically or colposcopically and then treat if the lesion is persistent or progressive after 18 to 24 months, and, if regression occurs, discharge her from the colposcopy clinic. In the context of developing countries, a decision may be made to treat the woman, as many fail return for a follow-up visit. If the decision is made to treat the woman with cryotherapy or LEEP, at least one follow-up visit should be scheduled at 9 to 12 months from the date of treatment (see Chapters 12 and 13). After cryotherapy and LEEP, healing of the cervix is grossly apparent by three to four weeks; cytological and colposcopic appearances will continue to reflect healing or regenerative effects for approximately three months. If the follow-up visit reveals no evidence of persistent disease, the woman can be discharged from the colposcopy clinic and advised to participate in the screening programme, if one is on-going in the region. Otherwise, she may be advised to undergo a repeat screening examination after three to five years. If persistent disease is found during the follow-up visit, appropriate investigations and appropriate treatment with cryotherapy, LEEP or cold-knife conization should be carried out.

Table 11.2: Indications for cold-knife conization

- The lesion extends into the endocervical canal and it is not possible to confirm the exact extent.

- The lesion extends into the canal and the farthest extent exceeds the excisional capability of the LEEP cone technique (maximum excisional depth of 1.5 cm).

- The lesion extends into the canal and the farthest extent exceeds the excisional capability of the colposcopist.

- The cytology is repeatedly abnormal, suggesting neoplasia, but there is no corresponding colposcopic abnormality of the cervix or vagina on which to perform biopsy.

- Cytology suggests a much more serious lesion than that which is seen and biopsy-confirmed.

- Cytology shows atypical glandular cells that suggest the possibility of glandular dysplasia or adenocarcinoma.

- Colposcopy suggests the possibility of glandular dysplasia or adenocarcinoma.

- Endocervical curettage reveals abnormal histology.

CIN 2-3

All women with high-grade lesions (CIN 2 or CIN 3) should be treated with cryotherapy or LEEP. They should strictly adhere to management protocols and be scheduled for a follow-up visit at 9 to 12 months after treatment (see Chapters 12 and 13). The woman can be discharged from the colposcopy clinic if the follow-up visit reveals no colposcopic or cytological evidence of persistent disease and she may be advised to resume participation in a screening programme, if one is on-going in the region, or may be followed up after three to five years. If persistent disease is found, the woman should receive appropriate treatment.

If a woman is treated with LEEP for any grade of CIN and the pathology report of a LEEP specimen indicates the possibility of an inadequate excision involving ectocervical or endocervical margins, she should be carefully evaluated in three follow-up visits with cytology, if available, and colposcopy, with special attention to the endocervical canal, at 3, 9 and 15 months. The problem of involved margins needs careful management. If persistent disease is found in any of these follow-up visits, the patient should be treated appropriately and followed up. If there is cytological, ECC or colposcopic evidence of a persistent lesion, and the limits can be seen and are within the range of a LEEP cone, then LEEP may be carried out. Otherwise, a cold-knife conization should be performed to ensure complete removal of the lesion. If the woman's results are normal in all three follow-up visits, she may re-enter a screening programme, or be followed up once in three or five years.

Invasive cancer

A diagnosis of invasive squamous cell carcinoma or adenocarcinoma requires prompt referral for definitive treatment with surgery and/or radiotherapy, with or without chemotherapy.

Women requiring further diagnostic investigations

Some cases assessed by colposcopy require more extensive diagnostic investigations before treatment. A mainstay in such investigation of women is cold-knife conization procedure. The indications for diagnostic cone biopsy are shown in Table 11.2. If the CIN lesion extends deep into the endocervical canal (i.e., more than 1.5 cm) or its upper limit is not visible, cold-knife conization is indicated. Women with any cytological report of an abnormality suggesting the possibility of

glandular dysplasia should have ECC performed in addition to colposcopic assessment. If ECC does not show evidence of a glandular lesion (but cytology does), cold-knife conization may be indicated. Women with cytology suggestive of adenocarcinoma or with histological evidence of glandular dysplasia or adenocarcinoma should have cold-knife conization to thoroughly evaluate the extent and severity of disease. If adenocarcinoma is found, it should be definitively treated as soon as possible.

Pregnant women

Pregnancy may be a woman's first opportunity to be screened for cervical cancer as part of routine prenatal care. In this case, she may often be referred for colposcopy following an abnormal cytology smear result before to the midpoint of the pregnancy. The usual scenarios and recommendations as to how each should be managed are discussed below.

Colposcopists should note that lesions seen in the cervix of a pregnant woman may become smaller post-partum due to shrinkage of the cervix. Lesions will tend to migrate post-partum towards the os due to inversion (the opposite of eversion) of the cervical epithelium. Therefore, a lesion followed into the post-partum period may appear smaller and may be located more into the canal than on the ectocervix.

During pregnancy, it is considered adequate management to base a working diagnosis on a colposcopic assessment of CIN without biopsy confirmation. If there is any slight doubt that the disease may be invasive cancer, a biopsy should be obtained. Since referral and colposcopic diagnosis usually occur near the midpoint of pregnancy, the woman in whom a high-grade CIN is suspected may be reviewed at about 28 weeks' gestation. Cytological and colposcopic examinations should be performed at both visits. If the cytological or colposcopic diagnosis changes to a more severe degree of abnormality at any of the follow-up visits during pregnancy, a directed punch biopsy should be obtained. If the disease is stable, the woman can be seen at two to three months post-partum for definitive diagnosis by biopsy and appropriate management of any lesion(s). The management plans for women at post-partum follow-up visits depend on the final diagnosis, and correspond to those described for nonpregnant women.

Vaginal delivery can be allowed if microinvasion or CIN is confirmed and definitive post-partum reassessment and treatment are planned. These women should be seen for definitive reassessment at 8 to 12 weeks post-partum. The cervix should be completely involuted and/or healed before re-colposcopy.

Treatment of cervical intraepithelial neoplasia by cryotherapy

- Cryotherapy and loop electrosurgical excision procedure (LEEP) are suitable and effective treatment options for CIN in both low- and high-resource settings, as both require less financial investment for equipment and maintenance, and both can be learnt in a short period of time.

- Compared to equipment required for LEEP, cryotherapy equipment costs substantially less.

- Cryotherapy relies on a steady supply of compressed refrigerant gases (N_2O or CO_2) in transportable cylinders. Cryotherapy is not adequate to treat lesions involving the endocervix.

- If excellent contact between the cryoprobe tip and the ectocervix is achieved, N_2O-based cryotherapy will achieve –89°C and CO_2-based system will achieve –68°C at the core of the ice ball and temperatures around –20°C at the edges. Cells reduced to –20°C for one or more minutes will undergo cryonecrosis.

- Healing takes place throughout the first six weeks after cryotherapy. Women may experience watery vaginal discharge for 3-4 weeks after treatment.

- Women should be advised not to use a vaginal douche, tampons or have sexual intercourse for one month after treatment.

- Cryotherapy may increase the transmissibility of HIV infection and using condoms is an effective means of prevention.

- Treatment failure is observed in about 5-10% of women.

Ablative and excisional treatments constitute two forms of out-patient surgical treatment of cervical intraepithelial neoplasia (CIN). Cryotherapy, electrocoagulation, cold coagulation and laser ablation are different methods of ablative treatment of CIN. The loop electrosurgical excision procedure (LEEP), using thin wire loop electrodes and long needle electrode electro-surgical cylindrical excision are the major forms of out-patient excisional treatment of CIN.

Of all available and effective treatments of CIN, cryotherapy and LEEP are appropriate for both high- and low-resource settings for several reasons and, hence, only these two methods are discussed in this field manual. First, they require the least financial investment for equipment, maintenance and repair. Second, once colposcopy has been mastered, cryotherapy and LEEP can be quickly learned and result in high cure rates and few complications. Other surgical techniques that are based on the laser or electrocoagulation are beyond the scope of this manual and the learner is referred to excellent books that have been written on their use (Wright *et al.*, 1992; Wright *et al.*, 1995; Singer & Monaghan, 2000).

The primary concern in treating CIN by ablative (destructive) or excisional techniques is whether the treatment will be adequate to eradicate any CIN that has extended down into the crypts underlying the neoplastic epithelium. The possible depth of crypt involvement increases with the severity of the CIN. A treatment that is effective to a depth of 7 mm is necessary to destroy CIN 3. The total linear extent of the lesion is also a factor to be considered. The linear extent of a lesion is the sum of its two distances, each measured from a reference point at the external os: the distance to the proximal edge (towards or into the canal) and the distance to the distal edge of the lesion (away from the canal). The average linear extent is 7.5 mm (range 2 to 22 mm) with 85 to 90% of lesions entirely visible externally on the transformation zone (Wright *et al.*, 1995). Vaginal extension is present in no more than 5% of patients.

The principles and practice of cryotherapy are discussed in this chapter and LEEP is described in the next chapter. Cryotherapy equipment (Figures 12.1, 12.2, and 12.3) costs substantially less to buy and to maintain than that required for LEEP. Cryotherapy does not require a source of electricity as LEEP does, but relies instead on a supply of easily transportable tanks of highly compressed refrigerant gas. After the vaginal speculum is in place and the cervix has been visualized, both procedures take approximately 15 minutes from start to finish.

Ancillary equipment is required for LEEP, but not for cryotherapy for several reasons. Although the performance of cryotherapy usually does not require a local anaesthetic, LEEP does require several injections of a local anaesthetic into the ectocervix. LEEP generates smoke that remains in the vagina unless it is evacuated by a vacuum system to allow an unobstructed view of the operative field. The third type of ancillary equipment required for LEEP is an electrically insulated vaginal speculum (and insulated vaginal side-wall retractor, if necessary) (Figure 13.3) or a metallic speculum insulated with latex condom (Figure 4.9) to prevent an electrical injury (shock or thermal injury) to the patient or the operator if the loop or the ball electrode accidentally touches the instrument. Since a metallic vaginal speculum conducts electricity, it may lead to an electrical injury to the vagina if the loop accidentally comes into contact with these metallic instruments. Insulated vaginal specula and insulated vaginal side-wall retractors are more expensive than non-insulated ones.

In contrast to LEEP, which is an excisional technique, cryotherapy is an ablative one. In practical terms, this means that there will be no pathology specimen to evaluate after cryotherapy which obviously has an immediate cost saving. Proponents of LEEP appreciate the feedback of information if there is a pathological examination of the LEEP excised tissue. This feedback allows a reassessment of not only the most severe grade of lesion present, but also the adequacy of excision (whether excisional margins are involved).

The main limitation of cryotherapy is that it is not adequate to treat lesions that are not wholly located on the ectocervix, yet involve the endocervical canal. In contrast, LEEP can adequately excise the majority of cervical lesions, whether or not the canal is involved. Meta-analysis of randomized clinical trials that evaluated the comparative effectiveness of cryotherapy with therapies such as LEEP, conization and laser, have concluded that the above treatments are equally effective in controlling CIN (Nuovo *et al.*, 2000; Martin-Hirch *et al.*, 2000). From the foregoing comparisons and contrasts, it is empirically clear that the most practical and cost-effective method of treatment of CIN in low-resource settings is cryotherapy, provided the lesion is wholly ectocervical in location. LEEP is the treatment of choice if the lesion involves the endocervical canal (see Chapter 13).

Since LEEP is technically more demanding than cryotherapy, we suggest that colposcopists should first demonstrate competence with cryotherapy before they perform LEEP.

If living tissue is frozen to a temperature of -20°C or lower for at least 1 minute, cryonecrosis ensues. Several features distinguish this process: intra- and extra-cellular crystallization, dehydration, thermal shock, vascular stasis and protein denaturation. A rapid freeze followed by a slow thaw is the most damaging to cells, especially neoplastic cells. A sequence of two freeze-thaw cycles (freeze-thaw-freeze-thaw) may produce more tissue destruction than a single cycle.

The cryotherapy technique uses a cryoprobe with a tip made of highly conductive metal (usually silver and copper), that makes direct surface contact with the ectocervical lesion. A substantial drop in temperature is achieved when a compressed refrigerant gas is allowed to expand through a small aperture in the cryoprobe. Nitrous oxide (N_2O) or carbon dioxide (CO_2) are the refrigerants of choice, as both provide excellent thermal transfer when circulating in the probe tip.

Cryotherapy equipment (Figures 12.1-12.4)

The cryotherapy unit consists of a compressed gas cylinder (tank), a yoke with a tightening knob and an inlet of gas to connect the gas cylinder to the

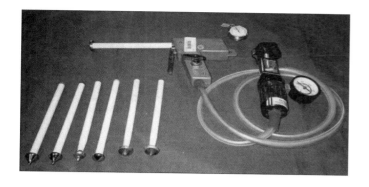

FIGURE 12.1: Cryoprobes, the cryogun, pressure gauge and stop watch

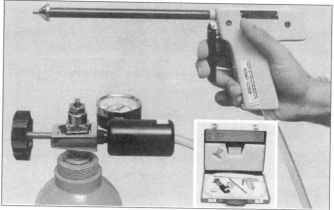

FIGURE 12.2: Cryotherapy equipment

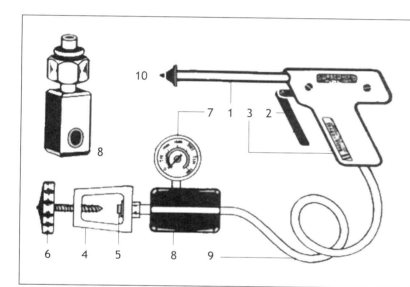

1. Probe
2. Trigger
3. Handle grip (fibreglass)
4. Yoke
5. Instrument inlet of gas from cylinder
6. Tightening knob
7. Pressure gauge showing cylinder pressure
8. Silencer (outlet)
9. Gas-conveying tube
10. Probe tip

FIGURE 12.3: Components of cryotherapy equipment

cryotherapy gun through a flexible gas-conveying tube, a pressure gauge showing the cylinder gas pressure, an outlet silencer, a cryotherapy gun with handle grip, a gas trigger to allow the gas to be released to the cryotherapy probe at high pressure and the cryotherapy probe. In most equipment, the pressure gauge shows three colour zones: yellow, green and red. When the gas cylinder is opened, if the pressure indicator in the gauge moves to the green zone, there is adequate gas pressure for treatment; if the needle remains in the yellow zone, the pressure is too low and the gas cylinder should be changed before commencing treatment; if the needle moves to the red zone, excess pressure is indicated and this excess pressure should be released. One should consult the manual provided by the manufacturer thoroughly for operational instructions.

Cryotherapy for ectocervical lesions

Eligibility criteria that must be met for cryotherapy are given in Table 12.1. If the woman is suffering from cervicitis, trichomoniasis or bacterial vaginosis, she may be offered a choice of having either cryotherapy immediately with simultaneous antimicrobial treatment or antimicrobial treatment and returning two to three weeks later for cryotherapy (see Chapter 11, Table 11.1). If there is evidence of pelvic inflammatory disease (PID), it is advisable to delay cryotherapy until the infection has been treated and resolved. If there is marked atrophy due to estrogen deficiency in an older woman and staining of the outer margin of a lesion is indistinct, cryotherapy may be carried out after a course of topical estrogen treatment and colposcopic reassessment. The woman must give written consent

Table 12.1: Eligibility criteria for cryotherapy

- The entire lesion is located in the ectocervix without extension to the vagina and/or endocervix

- The lesion is visible in its entire extent and does not extend more than 2 to 3 mm into the canal

- The lesion can be adequately covered by the largest available cryotherapy probe (2.5 cm); the lesion extends less than 2 mm beyond the cryotherapy probe

- CIN is confirmed by cervical biopsy/colposcopy

- There is no evidence of invasive cancer

- The endocervical canal is normal and there is no suggestion of glandular dysplasia

- The woman is not pregnant

- If the woman has recently delivered, she is at least three months post-partum

- There is no evidence of pelvic inflammatory disease

- The woman has given informed written consent to have the treatment

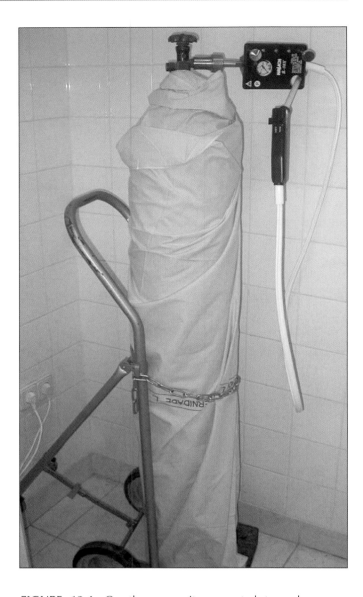

FIGURE 12.4: Cryotherapy unit connected to a large gas cylinder (covered with a clean cloth) which is safely placed on a moveable carrier

to have the treatment, after being thoroughly informed as to how it will be performed and the probabilities of its effectiveness, adverse effects, complications, long-term sequelae, and alternative ways that can be used to manage her problem.

It is advisable to use the largest cylinder of refrigerant gas possible, so that a sufficient amount of refrigerant is available to complete the treatment and the pressure forcing the refrigerant through the probe tip is maintained at a high level so that the effectiveness of the procedure is maintained. Standard-size tanks only allow adequate pressure to treat three women. A large tank has the advantage of treating more women, but transport from clinic to clinic may pose a problem.

If excellent contact is achieved between the probe tip and the ectocervix (Figures 12.5 and 12.6b), a nitrous oxide-based cryotherapy will achieve temperatures of about -89°C and the carbon dioxide-based system will achieve -68°C at the core of the tissue ice ball. The temperature at the edges of the frozen tissue may be around -20°C. Cells held at -20°C for one minute or more will undergo cryonecrosis. The minimum temperature at the probe tip for effective freezing should be -60°C. It is critical to establish and maintain good contact throughout the procedure between the probe tip and the tissue - poor contact means a relatively large variation in the temperatures achieved within the ice ball and therefore variable effectiveness in the target tissue.

The step-by-step approach to cryotherapy (Figures 12.5 and 12.6):

A woman should meet the eligibility criteria in Table 12.1. Generally, it is preferable to have the diagnosis of CIN firmly established before cryotherapy is performed. However, there may be exceptions to this general rule. For example, in developing countries, women may be offered treatment at their first colposcopy visit to maximize treatment coverage (otherwise patients lost to follow-up would not receive treatment for lesions) on the basis of a colposcopy diagnosis. However, directed biopsy may be carried out before instituting cryotherapy, so that a histological diagnosis will be available to establish the nature of the lesion treated a *posteriori*. The consequences of such an approach in terms of possible over-treatment or unnecessary treatment, as well as the side-effects and complications of the treatment procedure, should be explained and informed consent obtained.

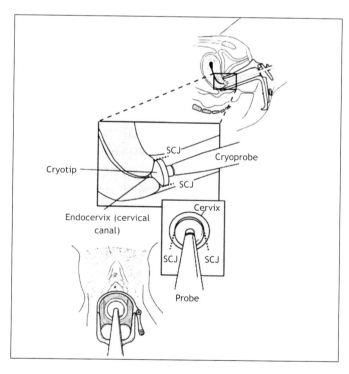

FIGURE 12.5: Positioning of the cryoprobe tip on the ectocervix

The provider should be familiar with the cryotherapy equipment and its different components (Figures 12.1-12.4) that will be used in a given setting. The instructions for operational use and safety provided by the manufacturer should be read carefully. The safety regulations should be strictly followed. Before cryotherapy is initiated, the gas tank pressure should be checked to ensure that it is sufficient to provide an effective flow of the refrigerant through the probe tip for the required duration of treatment. One should follow the instruction of the manufacturer in this regard. In most models of cryotherapy equipment, a green zone in the pressure gauge indicates adequate pressure (40-70 kg per cm^2) and a yellow zone indicates low pressure (less than 40 kg/cm^2). If there is adequate gas pressure in the cylinder, the indicator moves to the green zone in the gauge, after the cylinder is opened to release the gas. If the pressure is low, there will be insufficient freezing to give the required extent of cryonecrosis. The minimum working pressure shown on the gauge should be 40 kg/cm^2, and the freezing will be inadequate if the pressure falls below this level. In such an event, the gas cylinder should be changed before continuing treatment.

If the woman is returning to the clinic on a second visit (after histological confirmation) for treatment, colposcopic assessment should be done immediately before cryotherapy to confirm that the location and linear extent of the lesion are amenable to effective cryotherapy.

The physician or the nurse should explain the treatment procedure to the woman and reassure her. This is important to help the woman to relax during the procedure. After ensuring she has emptied her bladder, she should be placed in a modified lithotomy position and the cervix should be exposed with the largest speculum that can be introduced comfortably. The secretions are removed with a cotton swab soaked in saline. Then 5% acetic acid is applied and the cervix is examined with the colposcope. Following this, Lugol's iodine is applied to delineate the limits of the lesion. There is no need for local anaesthesia when performing cryotherapy.

The cryoprobe surface is wiped with saline to ensure adequate thermal contact with the cervix and optimal lowering of the tissue temperature. The cryotherapy probe tip is then firmly applied, with the centre of the tip on the os. It is obligatory to ensure that the vaginal walls are not in contact with the cryoprobe tip. The timer is then set and the gas trigger in the cryogun is released or squeezed to cool the cryoprobe in contact with the cervix. The gas escapes through the pressure gauge with a hissing noise. One should be able to observe ice being formed on the tip of the cryoprobe and on the cervix as freezing progresses. Make sure that the probe adequately covers the lesion and the tip does not inadvertently contact and freeze any part of the vagina during the procedure.

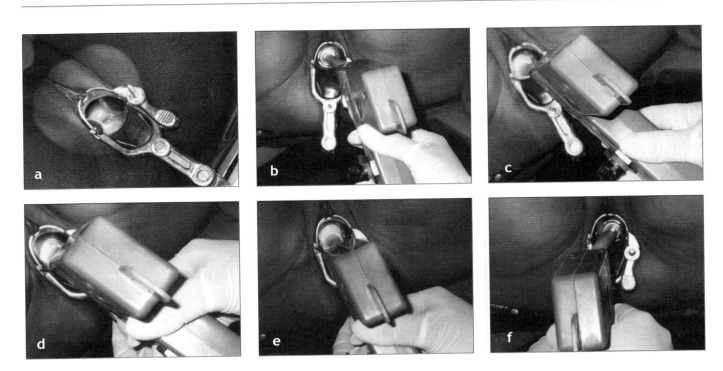

FIGURE 12.6: Cryofreezing in progress. Note the cryoprobe covers the lesion well (a, b). Note the iceball formation in c, d and e. Note the appearance after thawing in (f)

Cryotherapy should consist of two sequential freeze-thaw cycles, each cycle consisting of 3 minutes of freezing followed by 5 minutes of thawing (3 minutes freeze-5 minutes thaw-3 minutes freeze-thaw). The treatment time should be monitored using a stop watch. Adequate freezing has been achieved when the margin of the ice ball extends 4-5 mm past the outer edge of the cryotip. This will ensure that cryonecrosis occurs down to at least 5 mm depth. To achieve this effect evenly throughout the treatment field, it is extremely important to establish and maintain excellent contact between the probe tip and the ectocervical surface. Once the second freeze for 3 minutes is completed, allow time for adequate thawing before removing the probe from the cervix. When thawing is completed, the ice formation on the cryoprobe tip is totally cleared and the probe is removed by gently rotating on the cervix. Do not attempt to remove the probe tip from the cervix until complete thawing has occurred. After removing the probe, examine the cervix for any bleeding. The appearance of the cervix immediately after cryotherapy is shown in Figure 12.7a. Note the iceball formed in the cervix. The vagina should not be packed with gauze or cotton after cryotherapy to allow the secretions to escape. Women may be provided with a supply of sanitary pads to prevent the secretions staining their clothes.

After use, the probe tip should be wiped with 60-90% ethyl or isopropyl alcohol and then cleaned well with boiled water and disinfected with 2% glutaradehyde (see Chapter 14) and kept dry. After the procedure is completed, the cryogun, tubing, pressure gauge and gas tank should be de-contaminated by wiping with cotton soaked with 60-90% ethyl or isopropyl alcohol.

Follow-up after cryotherapy

Women should receive instructions on self-care and what symptoms to expect after treatment. They should be informed that they may experience some mild cramps and a clear or lightly blood-stained watery discharge for up to 4-6 weeks after treatment. Women should be advised not to use a vaginal douche or tampons or to have sexual intercourse for one month after treatment. They should be instructed to report if they have any one of the following symptoms in the six weeks after treatment: fever for more than two days, severe lower abdominal pain, foul-smelling- pus coloured discharge, bleeding with clots or bleeding for over two days. It is preferable to give written instructions on the above aspects and on follow-up.

Healing takes place during the first six weeks after cryotherapy. Granulation tissue is present in the wound during the first 2-3 weeks after cryotherapy (Figure 12.7b), which is followed by re-epithelialization of the

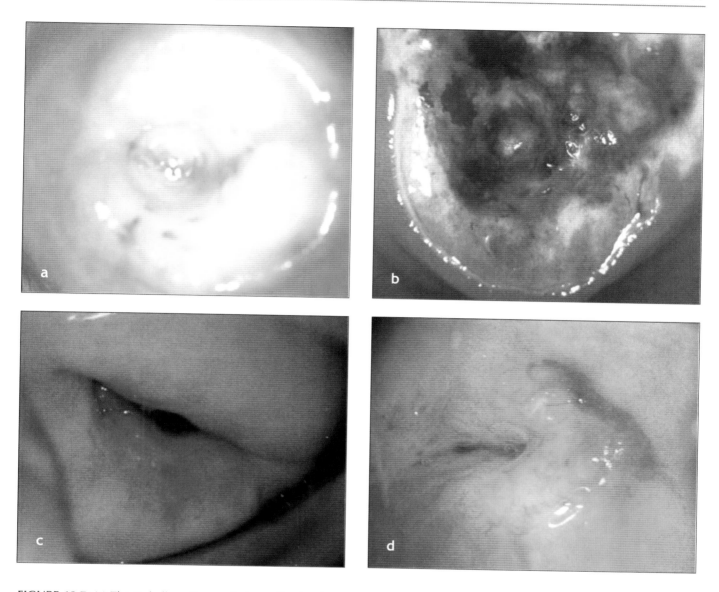

FIGURE 12.7: (a) The iceball on the cervix immediately after cryotherapy, (b) Appearance 2 weeks after cryotherapy. (c) 3 months after cryotherapy. (d) 1 year after cryotherapy

surface. Normally, the wound is totally healed within 6-8 weeks of treatment. The appearance of the cervix 3 months and 12 months after cryotherapy is shown in figures 12.7c and 12.7d.

The effect of cryotherapy on the potential transmissibility of human immunodeficiency virus (HIV) infection (to or from women) during the healing phase is not known. HIV-1 shedding in the vaginal secretions after treatment of CIN in HIV-positive women has been demonstrated (Wright *et al.*, 2001). Therefore, the authors suggest advising all women that cryotherapy may increase the transmissibility of HIV and that using condoms is an effective means of prevention. Condoms should be used for a period of at least four but preferably six weeks. Ideally, a supply of condoms should be available free of charge at colposcopy clinics in settings where HIV infection is endemic.

Appointments should be made for a follow-up visit 9-12 months after treatment. During the follow-up, cytology and/or VIA should be performed, followed by colposcopy and directed biopsy depending upon the colposcopy findings, to assess the regression or persistence of lesions. Retreatment is carried out if lesions persist. Women who are negative for neoplasia may be referred back to a screening programme (if one exists) or advised to undergo follow-up after three or five years.

Management of women for whom cryotherapy fails

Treatment failure is detected in about 5-10% of women

during the follow-up in the first year. These persistent, local or multifocal lesions are more likely to occur if the original lesion was large. To rule out the presence of unsuspected invasive carcinoma, it is advisable to biopsy all persistent lesions and then re-treat with cryotherapy, LEEP, or cold-knife conization, as appropriate. Follow-up evaluation may be carried out after 9-12 months in which screening examinations such as cytology and/or VIA and colposcopy should be carried out. Those negative for neoplasia may be referred back to a screening programme (if one exists in the region) or advised to undergo follow-up after three or five years. A management approach for low resource settings is shown in Figure 11.1.

Adverse effects, complications, and long-term sequelae

Cryotherapy is usually a painless procedure, if women have been properly reassured, their co-operation is obtained, and the procedure is carried out properly. Some women may experience some lower abdominal pain or cramps during and after cryotherapy. Once in a while, a woman may faint due to a vasovagal reaction. In such a situation, there is no need for panic and the women may be revived easily. Bleeding is extremely rare after cryotherapy.

Treated women experience a watery vaginal discharge for about 3-4 weeks after treatment. Vaginal bleeding is extremely unusual; it may be more likely to occur if freezing has been too aggressive and the ice ball has extended well past 5 mm in depth. The risk of post-operative infection is very slight and can probably be reduced further by delaying cryotherapy until any woman with a likely diagnosis of pelvic inflammatory disease (PID), sexually transmitted cervicitis (e.g., chlamydia or gonorrhea), vaginal trichomoniasis or bacterial vaginosis has been adequately treated and recovered. If a woman presents post-operatively with a malodorous discharge, pelvic pain and fever, the discharge may be cultured if possible, and empirical treatment should be prescribed with antibiotics that are effective for PID. Sexual partners should also be treated if the woman is diagnosed with PID, sexually transmitted cervicitis, or trichomoniasis. In developing countries, one may consider providing presumptive treatment with antibiotics routinely after cryotherapy (doxycycline 100 mg orally, two times a day, for seven days and metronidazole 400 mg orally, three times a day, for seven days).

Cervical stenosis occurs in less than 1% of women; reduced mucus production occurs in 5-10% of women. Cryotherapy has no known adverse effect on fertility and pregnancy. Invasive cancer has rarely been reported after cryotherapy, it is usually due to missed diagnosis as a result of poor diagnostic workup before cryotherapy.

Chapter 13

Treatment of cervical intraepithelial neoplasia by loop electrosurgical excision procedure (LEEP)

- Electrosurgical current applied to tissues can have one of three effects on the tissue, depending on the power setting and the waveform of the current used: desiccation, cutting, and fulguration.

- Loop electrosurgical excision procedure (LEEP) is a relatively simple procedure that can be readily learnt.

- The key advantage of LEEP over cryotherapy is that it removes rather than destroying the affected epithelium, allowing histological examination of the excised tissue.

- A loop wider than the lesion(s) and the transformation zone to be removed should be used; otherwise, the lesion should be removed with multiple passes.

- If the lesion involves the endocervical canal, a two-layer excisional method should be used.

- Women will have a brown or black discharge for up to two weeks after LEEP.

- Women should be advised not to use a vaginal douche, tampon, or have sexual intercourse for one month after LEEP.

- Moderate to severe post-operative bleeding occurs in less than 2% of treated women and they should be seen promptly.

- The failure rate with LEEP in women treated for the first time is around 10%.

Electrosurgery is the use of radiofrequency electric current to cut tissue or achieve haemostasis. A loop electrosurgical excision procedure (LEEP) operator needs to keep in mind that electricity flows to ground along the path of the least electrical resistance. The electrical energy used in electrosurgery is transformed into heat and light energy. The heat from a high-voltage electrical arc between the operating electrode and tissue allows the practitioner to cut by vaporizing tissue (at 100°C) or to coagulate by dehydrating tissue (above 100°C). The cutting electrodes are loops of very fine (0.2 mm) stainless steel or tungsten wire to achieve different widths, depths, and configurations of cut (Figure 13.1).

The higher temperatures involved in coagulation produce thermal effects greater than in electro-

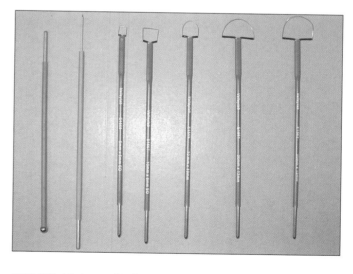

FIGURE 13.1: Ball electrode, macroneedle style electrode, loops

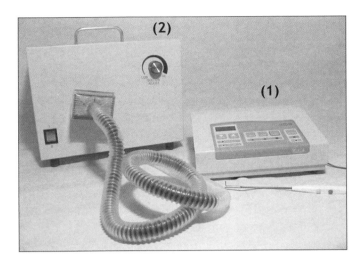

FIGURE 13.2: Electrosurgical generator (1) and the smoke evacuator (2)

surgical cutting. This is important in electrosurgery, since an adequate pathological examination requires that the coagulation effect be minimal in the excised surgical specimen. On the other hand, some coagulation effect is desirable, even while cutting, in order to minimize bleeding in the surgical field. Manufacturers of modern electrosurgical generators (Figure 13.2) are aware of the need to control bleeding. They offer electrosurgical cutting settings that lead to some coagulation by blending electrical currents, one with a cutting waveform and another with a coagulation waveform. This combination is called a blended cutting waveform, and is the type of waveform that will be referred to in this manual when electrosurgical cutting is discussed.

When the coagulation setting is selected on the electrosurgical generator, the coagulation waveform has a higher peak-to-peak voltage (producing higher temperatures) than that used for a pure cutting waveform, and is meant only to heat the tissue above 100°C to achieve dehydration. There are three types of coagulation: desiccation, in which the active electrode touches the tissue; fulguration, in which the active electrode does not touch the tissue but 'sprays' multiple sparks between itself and the tissue; and puncture coagulation, in which an electrode, usually a needle, is inserted into the centre of a lesion. Coagulation using the fulguration setting and a 3- to 5-mm ball electrode is the type of coagulation that is normally referred to in this manual (one exception is be the use of a needle electrode to fulgurate a stubborn area of bleeding). The fulguration setting uses a higher peak-to-peak voltage waveform than the

other coagulation settings, coagulating tissue with less current and, therefore, less potential harm to adjacent tissue.

To obtain a proper effect, an electrosurgical generator requires that a patient-return electrode or dispersive plate be used to allow the electrical circuit to be completed and the optimal current to flow. The dispersive plate should always be placed as close to the surgical site as possible. This is in contrast to the desired effect at the active electrode, where the current density is purposely high to concentrate the electrical energy as it is transformed into heat. Unless good electrical contact is maintained at the dispersive electrode over a large area, there is a danger that the patient will suffer from an electrical burn at this site. To guard against this possibility, modern electrosurgical units have circuitry (commonly referred to as a return electrode monitoring system) that continuously monitors the adequacy of the ground plate (dispersive pad) connection to the patient. This type of circuitry not only alerts the operator of a problem, but also prevents operation until the circuit fault is corrected. It is highly recommended that any electrosurgical generator meet the basic standards described above to ensure that safe and effective electrosurgery can be performed. It is assumed that only a system that meets or exceeds such requirements will be used in any of the electrosurgical procedures described in this manual.

Electrosurgery must not be performed in the presence of flammable gases, flammable anaesthetics, flammable liquids (e.g., alcohol-containing skin-preparation solutions or tinctures), flammable objects, oxidizing agents, or an oxygen-enriched atmosphere. The operator is, of course, at risk of receiving a burn from the active electrode if it is accidentally touched while activated.

Practising LEEP and demonstrating competence before use on patients

It is mandatory that every colposcopist has practised and demonstrated the ability to perform LEEP adequately by simulating the excision of cervical lesions on meat (beef, pork etc.) or fruits on which mock lesions have been painted to scale. Typewriter correction fluid or trichloroacetic acid work well for painting mock lesions. LEEP should always be practised using the colposcope, as is done in actual practice. If possible, colposcopists should have experience and demonstrated competence with cryotherapy before learning LEEP.

Table 13.1: The eligibiligy criteria that must be met before LEEP is performed

- CIN is confirmed by cervical biopsy, when possible

- If the lesion involves or extends into the endocervical canal, the distal or cranial limit of the lesion should be seen; the furthest (distal) extent is no more than 1 cm in depth

- There is no evidence of invasive cancer or glandular dysplasia

- There is no evidence of pelvic inflammatory disease (PID), cervicitis, vaginal trichomoniasis, bacterial vaginosis, anogenital ulcer or bleeding disorder

- If the woman has recently delivered, she should be at least three months post-partum

- Women with hypertension should have their blood pressure well controlled

- The woman must give written consent to have the treatment after being thoroughly informed as to how it is performed and the probabilities of its effectiveness, adverse effects, complications, long-term sequelae, and alternative ways that are available to manage her problem

The step-by-step approach to LEEP

First, it must be confirmed that the woman meets the eligibility criteria in Table 13.1.

If there is evidence of pelvic inflammatory disease (PID), cervicitis, vaginal trichomoniasis, bacterial vaginosis or anogenital ulcer, it is advisable to delay LEEP until that condition has been treated and resolved (see Chapter 11, Table 11.1). If there is marked atrophy due to estrogen deficiency in an older woman and staining of the outer margin of a lesion is indistinct, it is advisable to delay LEEP until after a course of topical estrogen treatment.

It is generally preferable to have the diagnosis of CIN firmly established before LEEP is performed. However, there may be exceptions to this general rule, for example, in the context of developing country settings, women may be offered treatment at their first colposcopy visit to maximize treatment coverage (otherwise patients lost to follow-up would not receive treatment for lesions). Expert colposcopists also may use this approach to maximize treatment coverage and to minimise the number of clinic visits in some clinical settings.

The instruments needed for LEEP should be placed on an instrument trolley or tray (Figure 13.3). If the woman is returning to the clinic on a second visit for treatment, colposcopic assessment should be carried out immediately before LEEP to confirm that the location and linear extent of the lesion are amenable to effective LEEP. The application of Lugol's iodine solution is helpful to outline lesion margins before the start of treatment. An insulated vaginal speculum (Figure 13.3) with an electrically insulating coating or a speculum covered with a latex condom (Figure 4.9) should be used to avoid an electrical shock to the woman in the event that the activated electrode inadvertently touches the speculum (though this type of event usually does not cause any tissue damage because of the relatively large area of contact). Similarly, care must be taken to avoid causing pain by inadvertently touching the vaginal walls with the activated electrode. The later possibility may be avoided by using an insulated vaginal sidewall retractor in addition to an insulated vaginal speculum (Figure 13.3) or by using a speculum covered by a condom (Figure 4.9).

It is ideal if the vaginal speculum used has a smoke evacuator tube attached to the luminal surface of the anterior blade so that a source of suction can be attached. If this type of speculum is not available, a simple suction tube (preferably made of non-conductive and non-flammable material) may be used, and the open tip should be positioned as near as possible to the cervix. A smoke evacuation system with a high rate of flow and a means of filtering out the smoke particles and odour is mandatory.

Local anaesthesia is achieved 30 seconds after multiple injections of a total of 5ml or less of 1% xylocaine (or a similar agent) into the stromal tissue of the ectocervix. The injections are given in a ring pattern 1-2 mm deep (at 3, 6, 9 and 12 o'clock

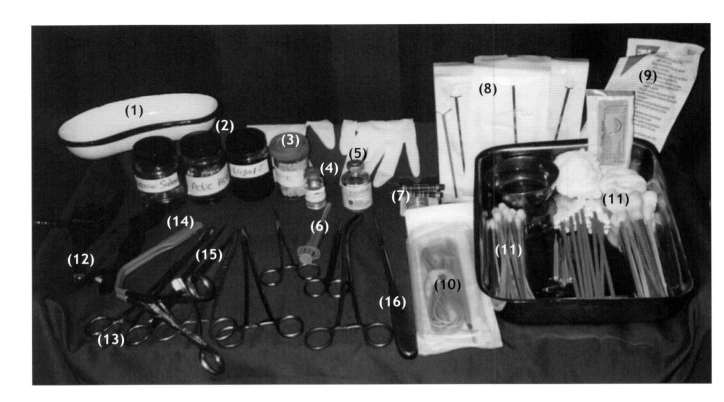

FIGURE 13.3: Instrument tray for LEEP

1: Kidney tray

2: Bottles with normal saline, 5% acetic acid and Lugol's iodine

3: Monsel's solution

4: Bottle containing formalin

5: Bottle containing local anaesthetic agent

6: Syringe for local anaesthesia

7: Needle and suture material

8: Loops and ball electrode

9: Patient return electrode or dispersive plate

10: Pencil with the hand switch

11: Cotton swabs

12: Insulated vaginal speculum

13: Sponge-holding forceps

14: Insulated vaginal side-wall retractor

15: Dissecting forceps

16: Endocervical curette

positions) at the periphery of the lesion and transformation zone using a 5ml syringe and 25- to 27-gauge needle. It is common practice to reduce the amount of bleeding during the procedure by mixing a vasoconstrictor agent such as vasopressin (no more than one pressor unit) with the injected local anaesthetic agent. The use of xylocaine with 2% adrenaline instead of pitressin also is adequate for local anaesthesia, but may cause palpitations and leg tremors before surgery. However, this can be avoided if infiltration is subepithelial. If a two-layer excision (LEEP cone) is planned, local anaesthetic is injected into the anterior and posterior endocervical canal also.

The aim of the LEEP procedure is to remove the lesions and the transformation zone in their entirety and send the affected tissue to the histopathological laboratory for examination. The least amount of power that will effectively perform the electrosurgery should be used, so as to minimize the risk to the patient's normal tissues and ensure that the excised specimen is in acceptable condition (with a minimum of thermal artifact) for pathological assessment. The power setting used depends on the size of the tissue electrode being used for cutting and whether fulguration is being performed - this information should be predetermined in each clinic and be available to the LEEP operator when choosing a power setting on the machine for cutting or fulguration. The commonly used power settings for the different loop electrodes are as follows: 1.0 x 1.0 cm 30 watts; 1.5 x 0.5 cm 35 watts; 2.0 x 0.8 cm 40 watts; 2.0 x 1.2 cm 50 watts. The power settings for 3 mm and 5 mm ball electrodes are 30 watts and 50 watts, respectively, in the coagulation mode. When possible, a lesion should be removed with one pass of the loop electrode, although this is not always feasible. Four basic operative scenarios are described below:

Excision of an ectocervical lesion with one pass (Figures 13.4 and 13.5)

The operator should use a loop that is wider than the lesion(s) and the transformation zone to be removed.

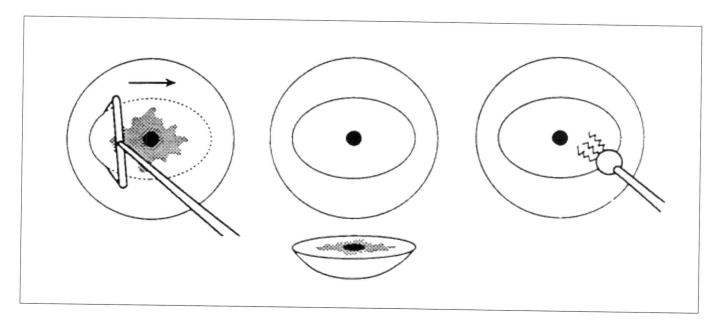

FIGURE 13.4: Excision of an ectocervical lesion with one pass

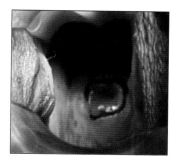 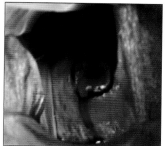 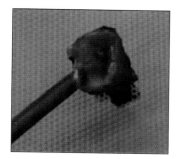 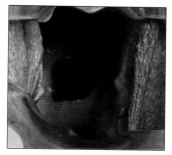

FIGURE 13.5: Excision of an ectocervical lesion with one pass. Note the excised specimen in place; the excised specimen is removed and the appearance of the cervix after the removal of the excised specimen.

The depth of the loop should be at least 5 mm (height from the cross bar to the farthest part of the wire arc). Often one may use a 2.0 x 0.8 cm oval loop. To maintain the ideal geometry and depth of cut, it is desirable to orient the surface of the ectocervix at right angles to the handle of the cutting electrode holder - that is, to keep the cross bar parallel to the ectocervix. To begin, local anaesthesia is administered, the electrosurgical generator is set to the appropriate power and blended cutting setting, and the smoke evacuation system is turned on. When the loop is poised just above the starting point, but not touching the cervical surface, the operator activates the current with a foot pedal or finger switch on the electrode holder. The loop is introduced into the tissue 5mm outside the outer boundary of the lesion. It is important not to push the electrode in, but to let it cut

its own way; the operator should simply provide directional guidance. The loop is directed gradually into the cervix until the cross bar nearly comes in contact with the epithelial surface. Then the loop is guided along parallel to the surface (horizontally or vertically, depending on the orientation of the direction of cutting) until the point is reached just outside the opposite border of the lesion. The loop is then withdrawn slowly, still keeping it at right angles to the surface. The current is switched off as soon as the loop exits the tissue. It does not matter whether the direction of excision is right to left or vice versa. It also is acceptable to pass the loop from the posterior to the anterior. However, it is not acceptable to pass the loop from the anterior to the posterior, since bleeding or excised tissue curling downward may obscure the visual field.

Once the specimen has been removed and placed in formalin, the setting on the electrosurgical generator is changed to fulguration and the appropriate power is selected. The surface of the excisional crater is fulgurated using 3 or 5 mm ball electrode, in the coagulation mode. The edges of the crater should also be fulgurated to preserve the squamocolumnar junction in the visible ectocervix. If active bleeding occurs and is difficult to control using the ball electrode, a macroneedle style electrode can be effectively used to apply the fulguration current in a much more concentrated (higher current density) and localized fashion to a bleeding site. If satisfactory haemostasis has been obtained, the surface of the crater is then coated with Monsel's paste and the speculum is removed. It is a general observation that an extremely nervous patient tends to bleed more than a relaxed one - another good reason to communicate with the patient throughout the procedure and to try to calm her fears.

If bleeding is difficult to stop despite use of the methods outlined above, the base of the excisional crater should be liberally coated with Monsel's paste and the vagina packed with gauze. The woman should be asked to wait for several hours before removing the pack. This complication appears to occur more frequently in women with cervicitis.

Excision of an ectocervical lesion with multiple passes (Figure 13.6)

If the diameter of a lesion exceeds the width of the largest loop (usually 2 cm), the lesion must be removed with multiple passes using one or more sizes of loop. Using the basic method described above (Figure 13.3), the central part of the lesion usually is removed first. The remaining parts of the lesion in the periphery are then removed by one or more separate passes. All specimens are preserved for pathological examination.

Excision of ectocervical plus endocervical lesions (Figures 13.7 and 13.8)

If a lesion involves the endocervical canal and is not likely to be removed with the depth of the usual single-layer pass as described above and shown in figures 13.4 and 13.5, a two-layer excisional method can be used. When lesions involve the canal, most of them extend for a linear length of 1 cm or less into the endocervical canal. Older women and women with CIN 3 are likely to have longer lesions and require a second layer - composed wholly of the endocervical canal - to be excised.

Usually the ectocervical portion of this type of lesion that extends into the canal can be excised by one pass of a large oval (2.0 x 0.8 cm) loop. The remaining tissue

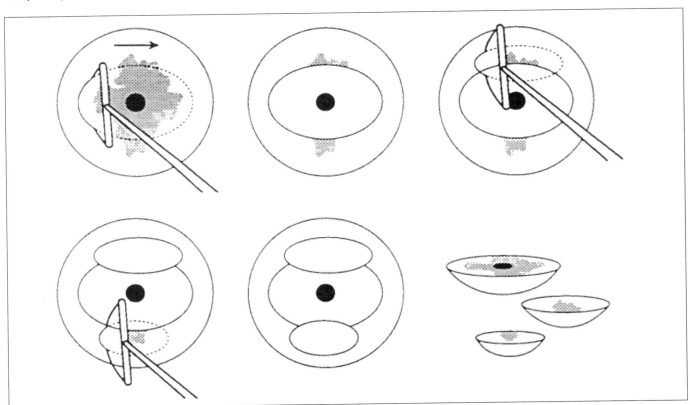

FIGURE 13.6: Excision of an ectocervical lesion with multiple passes

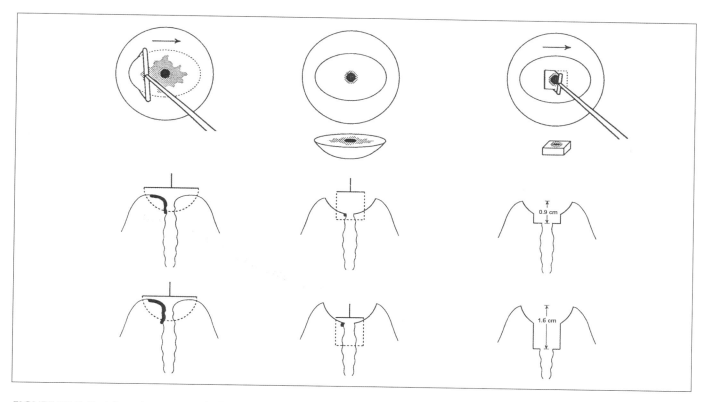

FIGURE 13.7: Excision of ectocervical plus endocervical lesions

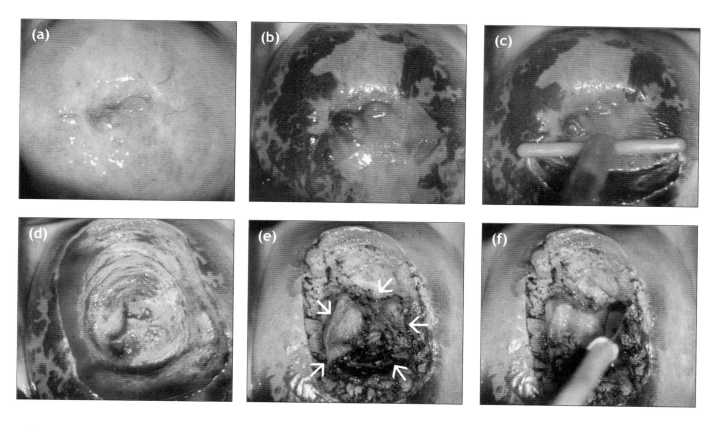

FIGURE 13.8: Excision of an ectocervical lesion extending into the endocervical canal by a two-layer excisional method; (a) appearance of the CIN 3 lesion after 5% acetic acid application; (b) appearance after Lugol's iodine application; (c) excision of the ectocervical lesion in progress; (d) ectocervical cut completed; (e) endocervical cut completed and the specimen in place (narrow arrows); (f) endocervical cut specimen removed and the bleeding points in the floor of the crater are being fulgurated to achieve haemostasis

in the endocervical canal can be excised using a smaller loop - usually a square loop with a 1.0 x 1.0 cm configuration - but care must be taken not to go any deeper than is necessary to completely excise the lesion and a margin of normal tissue. This type of excision can reach a maximum of 1.6 cm into the endocervical canal (Figure 13.7). Excision of this depth should be attempted only when absolutely necessary, due to increased risk of bleeding and stenosis as the depth of excision increases. LEEP should not be used if the distal or upper extent of the lesion in the canal cannot be seen and if the distal end of the lesion extends more than 1 cm into the canal. Such patients should undergo cold-knife conization. Since this two-step method requires adequate performance of the basic LEEP procedure, it is recommended that it should not be attempted until the operator is comfortable and competent with the basic LEEP. Women with lesions that extend further up into the canal need cold-knife conization to properly assess the endocervical canal.

Lesions with vaginal extension

If the lesion extends onto the vagina, it is preferable to use the ball electrode for electrofulguration on the peripheral, vaginal part of the lesion and LEEP on the central, cervical part of the lesion. The treatment of these vaginal lesions is beyond the scope of this manual and the LEEP treatment referred to here deals only with the type of lesions shown in Figures 13.4, 13.6, 13.7 and 13.8 and described above. Interested readers may refer to standard text books (Wright *et al.*, 1992; Wright *et al.*, 1995).

Follow-up care after LEEP

Women should receive instructions on self-care and what symptoms to expect after treatment. If appropriate, written instructions should be provided. Women should be advised that they will have a brown or black discharge lasting between a few days and two weeks. They should be advised to promptly report back if the discharge persists for more than two weeks, if discharge becomes malodorous and/or is associated with lower abdominal pain or if profuse bleeding develops. Women should be advised not to use a vaginal douche or tampons, or to have sexual intercourse for one month. The appearance of cervix three months and one year after LEEP is shown in Figures 13.9 and 13.10.

The effect of LEEP treatment on the potential transmissibility of HIV (to or from women) during the

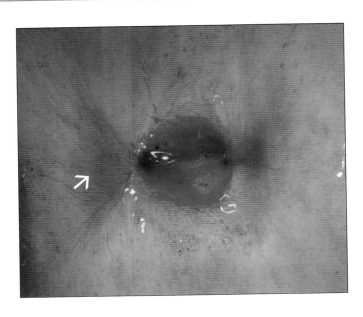

FIGURE 13.9: Appearance of the cervix three months after LEEP; note the parallel blood vessels in the healed cervix (arrow)

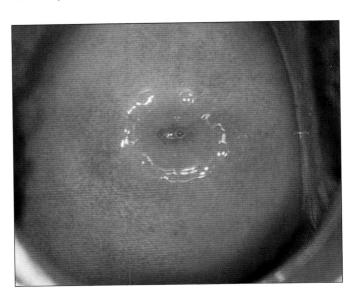

FIGURE 13.10: Appearance of the cervix one year after LEEP

healing phase is not known. HIV-1 shedding in the vaginal secretions after treatment of CIN in HIV-positive women has been demonstrated (Wright *et al.*, 2001). Therefore, the authors suggest advising all women that LEEP treatment may increase the transmissibility of HIV and that using condoms is an effective means of prevention. Condoms should be used for period of 6-8 weeks. Ideally, a supply of condoms should be available, free of charge, at colposcopy clinics in settings where HIV infection is endemic.

A follow-up appointment should be made for review at 9-12 months after treatment; the management plan should follow the scheme outlined in Chapter 11. Management of women who have persistent disease at the follow-up visit(s) is discussed in the next section.

Adverse effects, complications, and long-term sequelae of LEEP

Most women experience some transitory pain from the injection of local anaesthetic into the cervix. Severe perioperative bleeding occurs after 2% or less of LEEP procedures. Women should be advised to contact the clinic if they have any concerns during the post-operative period. It is advisable to give written post-operative instructions that outline the following points. Few women complain of post-operative pain. If post-operative pain occurs, it usually is similar to cramps; women should be instructed to use oral analgesics such as acetaminophen or ibuprofen, if necessary. A blood-tinged, dark brown (from the Monsel's paste) mucus discharge usually lasts for one or two weeks after treatment. Severe and moderate post-operative bleeding occurs in a few women, who should be seen promptly. Healing after LEEP usually takes place within a month.

When post-operative bleeding occurs, it usually appears 4-6 days after treatment and often from the posterior lip of cervix. This bleeding can usually be controlled by fulguration, applying Monsel's paste, or using a silver nitrate applicator stick. Rarely, placement of a suture at the bleeding site is necessary. The risk of post-operative infection is very small and can probably be reduced even more by delaying surgical treatment until any woman with a likely diagnosis of PID, cervicitis, vaginal trichomoniasis or bacterial vaginosis has been adequately treated and recovered. If a woman presents post-operatively with a malodorous discharge, it should be cultured if possible and empirical treatment prescribed with antibiotics that are effective for PID (see Table 11.1). In developing countries, it may be preferable to institute routine presumptive treatment with antibiotics after LEEP (doxycycline 100 mg orally, two times a day, for seven days and metronidazole 400 mg orally, three times a day, for seven days).

The squamocolumnar junction is in the endocervical canal at the follow-up evaluation in approximately 2% of women. This presents a challenge for adequate colposcopic examination and cytological sampling. Women should be warned that cervical stenosis, partial or complete, is rarely encountered (probably less than 1%), but is more common in menopausal women.

Management of women with persistent lesions at follow-up

All women, regardless of whether or not the pathology report states that the excisional margins are clear, should be followed up at 9 - 12 months from treatment to evaluate regression or persistence of lesions and complications. Treatment failures (persistent lesion(s) at follow-up) are detected in less than 10% of women when they are checked at the follow-up appointment. It is advisable to biopsy all persistent lesions to rule out the presence of unsuspected invasive carcinoma. Persistent lesions should be re-treated with cryotherapy or LEEP or cold-knife conization, as appropriate.

Chapter 14

Decontamination, cleaning, high-level disinfection and sterilization of instruments used during the diagnosis and treatment of cervical neoplasia

- Decontamination refers to steps taken to ensure that a medical instrument is safe for handling by reducing its contamination with microorganisms. This step results in the inactivation of hepatitis B virus and HIV.

- Cleaning ensures the removal of biological material from the instruments.

- The destruction of all micro-organisms, including bacterial spores on an instrument, is referred to as sterilization.

- When sterilization equipment is not available, or the instrument cannot be sterilized, high-level disinfection (HLD) is used. HLD results in all forms of microbes, except bacterial spores, being destroyed.

- Strict implementation of the above procedures according to a written manual is helpful in quality assurance of safe utilization of reusable instruments.

The basic steps involved in the safe utilization of reusable instruments for colposcopy and treatment of cervical intraepithelial neoplasia (CIN) are summarized in this chapter. A thorough knowledge and understanding of the steps in the high-level disinfection (HLD)/sterilization process is absolutely essential, as it ensures that the instruments used are free of infectious agents. Any lack of compliance with this process can lead to contamination of the sterilized instruments and harm to the patient. The process for re-use of the instruments begins with decontamination and continues through cleaning, sterilization/HLD, storage and handling. A quality assurance programme will help to ensure that instruments are processed adequately for re-use.

There are three basic steps before instruments, used for clinical and surgical procedures, can be reused: decontamination, cleaning and sterilization/HLD. These are briefly discussed and the methods used for sterilizing different instruments are described.

Decontamination

Decontamination comprises a series of steps to make a medical instrument or device safe for handling by reducing its contamination with microorganisms or other harmful substances. Usually, these procedures are performed by the nursing, technical or cleaning staff, and decontamination protects these workers from inadvertent infection. If these procedures are carried out properly, decontamination of the instruments will be assured before handling for cleaning. This step results in the inactivation of most organisms such as hepatitis B and HIV. Further processing is necessary to ensure that the object is cleaned and then sterilized.

Cleaning

Cleaning is a crucial step in providing safe, infection-free instruments. Vigorous manual cleaning with running water and liquid soap or detergent removes biological material such as blood, body fluids and tissue remnants. Instruments should be cleaned as soon as possible after use. If biological material is left behind, it can act as a sanctuary for residual microorganisms, protecting them from the effects of disinfection and sterilization.

Sterilization or high-level disinfection (HLD)

Sterilization is defined as the process of destroying all microorganisms on an instrument by exposure to physical or chemical agents. This process kills all forms of microbial life including bacterial spores. In practice, sterility is considered to be achieved if the probability of a surviving microorganism is less than one in a million. The sterilization process is fundamental for the safe reuse of instruments in clinical care.

When sterilization equipment is not available, or the instrument cannot be sterilized, HLD is used. Disinfection implies that the microbial burden of an instrument is reduced, but not entirely eliminated. The extent of this reduction depends upon the disinfection process used and the resistance of the microbial forms present. In practice, however, HLD results in all forms of microbial life being destroyed except bacterial spores.

Method of decontamination

Immediately after use, place instruments and other items, such as gloves, in a clean large plastic bucket containing 0.5% chlorine solution for 10 minutes. The 0.5% chlorine solution can be prepared by adding one part of concentrated household bleach (sodium hypochlorite solution, 5% available chlorine) to nine parts of water.

The general formula for making a dilute solution from a commercial preparation of any given concentration is as follows: Total parts of water = [% concentrate/% dilute] -1. For example, to make a 0.5% dilute solution of chlorine from 5% concentrated liquid household bleach = [5.0%/0.5%] -1 = 10-1 = 9 parts of water; hence add one part of concentrated bleach to nine parts of water.

If one is using commercially available dry powder chlorine, use the following formula to calculate the amount (in grams) of dry powder required to make 0.5% chlorine solution:

Grams/litre = [% dilute/% concentrate] x 1000.

For example to make a 0.5% dilute chlorine solution from a dry powder of 35% calcium hypochlorite = [0.5%/35%] x 1000 = 14.2 g. Hence add 14.2 grams of dry powder to 1 litre of water or 142 grams to 10 litres of water. The instruments should not be left in dilute bleach for more than 10 minutes and should be cleaned in boiled water immediately after decontamination to prevent discolouration and corrosion of metal.

Method of cleaning

Thorough manual cleaning of instruments with water and detergent to remove all organic material, after decontamination in 0.5% chlorine solution for 10 minutes, is of the utmost importance before to sterilization or HLD. A brush should be used to scrub the instruments free of biological matter. Instruments should be cleaned as soon as possible after use, so that no organic material will dry and stick to the instruments, providing a sanctuary for microbes. The person cleaning should use utility gloves while washing instruments.

Protective glasses or goggles should be worn by the cleaners to protect their eyes from contaminated water. Special attention should be given to instruments with teeth (e.g., biopsy punches), joints and screws (e.g., vaginal specula), to which biological material can become stuck. After cleaning, rinse the instruments thoroughly with boiled water to remove detergent residue.

Methods of sterilization

Instruments that are considered 'critical' (instruments entering sterile body tissues or vascular system, see Table 14.1, e.g. biopsy punch, surgical instruments, electrocautery tip, vaginal specula) require sterilization before re-use. Two methods of sterilization are described here.

(a) *High-pressure saturated steam sterilization* using autoclaves is recommended for sterilization. Unwrapped instruments should be exposed for 20 minutes to temperatures between 121-132°C at a pressure of 106 kPa (15 lb/inch^2). You should follow the manufacturer's advice, as pressure settings may vary slightly depending on the make of the autoclave. Small wrapped packs of instruments should be exposed for 30 minutes. The material used for wrapping should be porous enough to let steam through. Wrapped sterile instruments have a shelf life of up to seven days, if kept dry and intact. Unwrapped instruments should be placed in a sterile container. Small autoclaves are ideal for use in clinics.

(b) *Chemical sterilization* by soaking in 2-4% glutaraldehyde for 8 to 10 hours or 24 hours in 8% formaldehyde is an alternative to steam sterilization. This requires special handling with gloves, and the instruments thus sterilized should be rinsed with sterile water before use, as these chemicals form a residue on the instruments. Glutaraldehyde is very expensive, while formaldehyde is more irritating to skin, lung and eyes. Steam sterilization is preferred to chemical sterilization.

Methods of high-level disinfection (HLD)

Two methods of HLD are described here:

(a) Boiling plain tap water in a clean vessel offers a cheap and readily accessible form of HLD. The contact time for instruments should be at least 20 minutes after boiling has started. Water in the vessel should be changed daily. The vessel should be washed and kept dry every day.

(b) Alternatively, HLD may be obtained by soaking instruments in one of the following solutions for 20-30 minutes:

• *0.1% Chlorine solution:* If boiled water is used to make the solution, 0.1% chlorine may be used for HLD. If not, one should use 0.5% solution. The contact time required is 20 minutes. The solution is very corrosive to stainless steel. After disinfection, instruments should be thoroughly rinsed with boiled water and then air-dried or dried with a sterile cloth before use. The shelf life of prepared solution is one week.

• *6% Hydrogen peroxide solution:* It can be prepared by adding one part of a 30% solution to four parts of boiled water; the contact time is 30 minutes. After disinfection, instruments should be thoroughly rinsed with boiled water and then air-dried or dried with a sterile cloth before use. However, this solution will damage the external surfaces of rubbers and plastics, and corrode copper, zinc, and brass instruments after prolonged use.

• *2% Glutaraldehyde:* It must be prepared according to the manufacturer's instructions; activated 2% solution in a covered container has a shelf life of two weeks. The contact time is 20 minutes. As glutaraldehyde forms a residue on instruments, which is toxic to tissues, the instruments must be rinsed thoroughly with sterile water and dried with a sterile cloth before use.

Quality assurance

Strict implementation of decontamination, cleaning, and sterilization or HLD of instruments, according to a written manual is helpful in quality assurance of the procedures. The manual must be prominently displayed in the clinic for ready reference. The quality assurance process includes regular audits, analysis, system adjustments and education. The audits should include review of the methods of sterilization used, the items being sterilized, the length and temperature of exposure, identification of the person performing the sterilization, and periodic review and inspection of equipment being used for sterilization. The frequency of pelvic infection following clinical procedures in this context (i.e., screening, early detection and treatment of cervical pre-cancer) is a good indicator of the quality of sterilization process in place.

Spaulding's classification of medical instruments (modified)

Spaulding categorized medical instruments as 'critical', 'semi-critical', or 'non-critical', according to how they are used (Table 14.1). This is useful in guiding their processing for reuse.

Table 14.1: Spaulding's categorization of medical instruments

Class	Use	Processing
Critical, 'C'	Enters sterile body site or vascular system	Decontamination, cleaning followed by sterilization
Semi-critical, 'SC'	Comes into contact with intact mucous membrane or non-intact skin	Decontamination, cleaning followed by high-level disinfection (HLD)
Non-critical, 'NC'	Comes into contact with intact skin	Decontamination, cleaning followed by intermediate-level or low-level disinfection

Intermediate-level disinfection results in destruction of *Mycobacterium tuberculosis*, vegetative bacteria, most viruses (HIV, hepatitis B and herpes Simplex viruses) and most fungi (Candida, Aspergillus), but does not kill bacterial spores. Low-level disinfection destroys most bacteria, some viruses, some fungi, but not *Mycobacterium tuberculosis* or bacterial spores. 60-90% ethyl or isopropyl alcohol or iodophors such as 10% povidone iodine act as intermediate or low-level disinfectants. While alcohol does not leave a residue on instruments, iodophors do. A guide to the processing of instruments and materials used for screening of cervical neoplasia, colposcopy and treatment of CIN is given in Table 14.2.

Decontamination of surfaces in the screening clinic

Procedure tables, trolleys, equipment (colposcope, cryosurgical equipment, electrosurgical generator, smoke evacuator, halogen lamp, etc.) in the screening clinic may be contaminated with body fluids such as vaginal secretions, purulent discharge, blood, etc. While the surface of the procedure table should be decontaminated after each patient procedure, the other surfaces should be decontaminated on a daily basis by wiping with 0.5% chlorine solution, 60-90% ethyl or isopropyl alcohol or other chemical disinfectants such as iodophors. The floor of the screening clinic should also be decontaminated on a daily basis.

Table 14.2: A guide to the processing instruments and materials used for early detection and treatment of cervical neoplasia

Instrument/material	Category	Processing	Suggested procedure
Vaginal speculum, vaginal retractors, biopsy forceps, endocervical curette, endocervical speculum, needle holder, toothed forceps, mosquito, vulsellum, forceps, insulated speculum and vaginal side-wall retractor	'C'	Decontamination and cleaning followed by sterilization or HLD	Autoclaving or disinfection with boiling water
Gloves	'C'	Decontamination and cleaning followed by sterilization	Autoclaving as wrapped packs
Cryoprobes	'SC'	Decontamination and cleaning followed by HLD	Disinfection with 0.1% chlorine or 2% glutaraldehyde or 6% hydrogen peroxide
Colposcope head, stand LEEP equipment, cryogun and regulator, cryo gas cylinder, examination table, hand lens, aviscope, torch lights, halogen lamp, instrument trolley, trays	'SC'	Intermediate or low-level disinfection	Wipe with 60-90% ethyl, isopropyl alcohol

C: Critical; SC: Semi-critical; NC: Non-critical; HLD: High-level disinfection

References

Anderson, M., Jordan, J., Morse, A., & Sharp, F. (1996) *Integrated Colposcopy*. 2nd ed. London and New York: Chapman Hall Medical.

Belinson, J.L., Pretorius, R.G., Zhang, W.H., Wu, L.Y., Qiao, Y.L. & Elson, P. (2001) Cervical cancer screening by simple visual inspection after acetic acid. *Obstet. Gynecol.*, **98**, 441-444.

Bosch, F.X., Manos, M.M., Muñoz, N., Sherman, M., Jansen, A.M., Peto, J., Schiffman, M.H., Moreno,V., Kurman, R., & Shah, K.V. (1995) The IBSCC Study Group. Prevalence of human papillomavirus in cervical cancer: a worlwide perspective. *J. Natl. Cancer. Inst.*, **78**, 796-802.

Broders, A.C. (1932) Carcinoma in situ contrasted with benign penetrating epithelium. *J. Am. Med. Assoc.*, **99**, 1670.

Burghardt, E., Baltzer, J., Tulusan, A.H., & Haas, J. (1992) Results of surgical treatment of 1028 cervical patients studied with volumetry. *Cancer*, **70**, 648-655.

Burghardt, E., Pickel, H., & Girardi, F. (1998) *Colposcopy Cervical Pathology. Textbook and Atlas*. Thieme, New York.

Campion, M., Feris, D., di Paola, F., & Reid, R. (1991) *Modern colposcopy - A practical approach*. Augusta. Educational System Inc.

Cartier R., & Cartier, I. (1993) *Practical Colposcopy*. 3rd edition. Paris: Laboratoire Cartier.

Coppleson, M., Reid, B., & Pixley, E. (1986) *Colposcopy*, 3rd Edition, Charles C Thomas, Springfield.

Coppleson, M. (1992) Early invasive squamous and adenocarcinoma of the cervix (FIGO stage 1a): clinical features and management. In: Coppleson, M. (ed) *Gynaecological Oncology*, Vol 1. 2nd edition, Churchill Livingston, Edinburgh.

Coppleson, M., Dalrymple, J.C., & Atkinson, K.H. (1993a) Colposcopic differentiation of abnormalities arising in the transformation zone. *Obstetrics and Gynecology Clinics of North America*, **20**, 83-110.

Coppleson, M., Dalrymple, J.C., & Atkinson, K.H. (1993b) Colposcopic differentiation of abnormalities arising in the transformation zone. In Wright, V.C. (Ed). *Contemporary Colposcopy*. Philadelphia: WB Saunders.

Delgado, G., Bundy, B., Zaino, R., Sevin, B.U., Creasman, W.T., & Major, F. (1990) Prospective surgical pathologic study of disease-free interval in patients with stage IB squamous cell carcinoma of the cervix: a Gynecologic Oncology Group study. *Gynecol. Oncol .*, **38**, 352-357.

Denny, L., Kuhn, L., Pollack, A., Wainwright, H., & Wright, T.C. Jr. (2000) Evaluation of alternative methods of cervical cancer screening for resource-poor settings. *Cancer*, **89**, 826-33.

Denton, A.S, Bond, S.J, Matthews, S., Bentzen, S.M., & Maher, E.J. (2000) National audit of the management and outcome of carcinoma of the cervix treated with radiotherapy in 1993. *Clin. Oncol. (R. Coll. Radiol.)*, **12**, 347-353.

Fagundes, H., Perez, C.A., Grigsby, P.W., & Lockett, M.A. (1992) Distant metastases after irradiation alone in carcinoma of the uterine cervix. *Int. J. Radiat. Oncol. Biol. Phys.*, **24**, 197-204.

Ferenczy, A., & Franco, E. (2002) Persistent human papillomavirus infection and cervical neoplasia. *Lancet Oncol.*, **3**, 11-16.

Franco, E.L., Rohan, T.E., & Villa, L.L. (1999) Epidemiologic evidence and human papillomavirus infection as a necessary cause of cervical cancer. *J. Natl. Cancer Inst.*, **91**, 506-511.

Franco, E.L., Villa, L.L., Sobrino, J.P., Prado, J.M., Rousseau, M.C., Desy, M., & Rohan, T.E. (1999) Epidemiology of acquisition and clearance of cervical human papillomavirus infection in women from a high-risk area for cervical cancer. *J Infect. Dis.*, **180**, 1415-1423.

Gatta, G., Lasota, M.B., & Verdecchia, A. (1998) Survival of European women with gynaecological tumours, during the period 1978-1989. EUROCARE Working Group. *Eur. J. Cancer*, **34**, 2218-2225.

Green, J.A, Kirwan, J.M., Tierney, J.F, Symonds, P., Fresco, L., Collingwood, M., & Williams, C.J. (2001) Survival and recurrence after concomitant chemotherapy and radiotherapy for cancer of the uterine cervix: a systematic review and meta-analysis. *Lancet*, **358**, 781-786.

Herrero, R., Schiffman, M.H., Bratti, C., Ildesheim, A., Balmaceda, I., Sherman, M.E., Greenberg, M., Cardenas, F., Gomez, V., Helgesen, K., Morales, J., Hutchinson, M., Mango, L., Alfaro, M., Potischman, N.W., Wacholder, S., Swanson, C., & Brinton, L.A. (1997) Design and methods of a population-based natural history study of cervical neoplasia in a rural province of Costa Rica: the Guanacaste project. *Pan. Am. J. Public Health*, **1**, 362-375.

Herrero, R. (1997) Prevalence surveys of HPV infection in high- and low-incidence areas for cervical cancer. In: *International Agency for Research on Cancer-Biennial report 1996/1997*. Lyon, France: IARC press, 68-69.

Hinselmann, H. (1925) Verbesserung der Inspektionsmoglichkeiten von Vulva, Vagina and Portio. *Munchner Med Wochenschr*, **72**, 1733-42.

Ho, G.Y, Bierman, R., Beardsley, L., Chang, C.J., & Burk, R.D. (1998) Natural history of cervicovaginal papillomavirus infection in young women. *N. Engl. J. Med.*, **338**, 423-428.

Ho, G.Y., Burk, R.D., Klein, S., Kadish, A.S., Chang, C.J., Palan, P., Basu, J., Tachezy, R., Lewis, R., & Romney, S. (1995) Persistent genital human papillomavirus infection as a risk factor for persistent cervical dysplasia. *J. Natl. Cancer Inst.*, **87**, 1365-1371.

Holowaty, P., Miller, A.B., & Rohan, T. (1999) Natural history of dysplasia of the uterine cervix. *J. Natl. Cancer Inst.*, **91**, 252-258.

Howard, M., Sellors, J., & Lytwyn, A. (2002) Cervical intraepithelial neoplasia in women presenting with external genital warts. *CMAJ*, **166**, 598-599.

IARC Working Group. (1995) *Human papillomaviruses. IARC Monograph on the evaluation of carcinogenic risks to humans*. Vol. 65. Lyon, France: International Agency for Research on Cancer.

Koutsky, L.A., Holmes, K.K., Critchlow, C.W., Stevens, C.E., Paavonen, J., Beckmann, A.M., DeRouen, T.A., Galloway, D.A., Vernon, D., & Kiviat, N.B. (1992) A cohort study of the risk of cervical intraepithelial neoplasia grade 2 or 3 in relation to papillomavirus infection. *N. Engl. J. Med.*, **327**, 1272-1278

Kosary, C.L. (1994) FIGO stage, histology,histologic grade, age and race as prognostic factors in determining survival for cancers of the female gynecological system: an analysis of 1973-87 SEER cases of cancers of the endometrium, cervix, ovary, vulva, and vagina. *Semin. Surg. Oncol.*, **10**, 31-46.

Kurman, R.J., Malkasian, G.D. Jr, Sedlis, A., & Solomon, D. (1991) From Papanicolaou to Bethesda: the rationale for a new cervical cytologic classification. *Obstet. Gynecol.*, **77**, 779-782.

Liaw, K.L., Glass, A.G., Manos, M.M., Greer, C.E., Scott, D.R., Sherman, M., Burk, R.D., Kurman, R.J., Wacholder, S., Rush, B.B., Cadell, D.M., Lawlerm, P., Tabor, D., & Schiffman, M. (1999) Detection of human papillomavirus DNA in cytologically normal women and subsequent cervical squamous intraepithelial lesions. *J. Nat.l Cancer Inst.*, **91**, 954-960.

Liaw, K.L., Hildesheim, A., Burk, R.D., Gravitt, P., Wacholder, S., Manos, M.M., Scott, D.R., Sherman, M.E., Kurman, R.J., Glass, A.G., Anderson, S.M., & Schiffman, M. (2001) A prospective study of human papillomavirus (HPV) type 16 DNA detection by polymerase chain reaction and its association with acquisition and persistence of other HPV types. *J. Infect. Dis.*, **183**, 8-15.

Martin-Hirsch, P.L., Paraskevaidis, E., & Kitchener, H. (2000) Surgery for cervical intraepithelial neoplasia. *Cochrane Database Syst. Rev.*, **2**, CD001318.

McIndoe, W.A., McLean, M.R., Jones, R.W., & Mullins, P.R. (1984) The invasive potential of carcinoma in situ of the cervix. *Obstet. Gynecol.*, **64**, 451-458.

Melnikow, J., Nuovo, J., Willan, A.R., Chan, B.K., & Howell, L.P. (1998) Natural history of cervical squamous intraepithelial lesions: a meta-analysis. *Obstet Gynecol.*, **92(4 Pt 2)**, 727-735.

Mitchell, M.F., Hittelman, W.N., Hong, W.K., Lotan, R., & Schottenfeld, D. (1994) The natural history of cervical intraepithelial neoplasia: an argument for intermediate endpoint biomarkers. *Cancer Epidemiol. Biomarkers Prev.*, **3**, 619-626.

Mitchell, M.F., Schottenfeld, D., Tortolero-Luna, G., Cantor, S.B., & Richards-Kortum, R. (1998) Colposcopy for the diagnosis of squamous intraepithelial lesions: Meta-analysis. *Obstet. Gynaecol.*, **91**, 626-31.

Moscicki, A.B., Hills, N., Shiboski, S., Powell, K., Jay, N., Hanson, E., Miller, S., Clayton, L., Farhat, S., Broering, J., Darragh, T., & Palefsky, J. (2001) Risks for incident human papillomavirus infection and low grade squamous intraepithelial lesion development in young females. *JAMA*, **285**, 2995-3002.

Moscicki, A.B., Shiboski, S., Broering, J., Powell, K., Clayton, L., Jay, N., Darragh, T.M., Brescia, R., Kanowitz, S., Miller, S.B., Stone, J., Hanson, E., & Palefsky, J. (1998) The natural history of human papillomavirus infection as measured by repeated DNA testing in adolescent and young women. *J. Pediatr.*, **132**, 277-284.

National Cancer Institute Workshop. (1989) The 1988 Bethesda System for reporting cervical/vaginal cytologic diagnoses. *JAMA*, **262**, 931-934.

National Cancer Institute Workshop. (1993) The Bethesda System for reporting cervical/vaginal cytologic diagnoses: revised after the second National Cancer Institute Workshop, April 29-30, 1991. *Acta Cytol.*, **37**, 115-124.

Nuovo, J., Melnikov, J., Willan, A.R., & Chan, N.K. (2000) Treatment outcomes for squamous intraepithelial lesions. *Int. J. Gynaecol. Obstet.*, **68**, 25-33.

Östor, A.G. (1993) Natural history of cervical intraepithelial neoplasia : a critical review. *Int J Gynecol. Pathol.*, **12**, 186-192.

Popkin, D.R. (1995) Pitfalls in colposcopy. In: Cecil Wright V, Likrish GM, & Shier RM (Eds). *Basic and advanced colposcopy. Part one: A practical handbook for diagnosis*. Second edition. Houston. Biomedical Communications.

Reagan, J.W., Seidermann, I.L., & Saracusa, Y. (1953) The cellular morphology of carcinoma in situ and dysplasia or atypical hyperplasia of the uterine cervix. *Cancer*, **6**, 224-235.

Reid, R. (1987) A rapid method for improving colposcopic accuracy. *Colposcopic and Gynaecologic Laser Surgery*, **3**, 139-146 .

Reid, R. (1993) Biology and colposcopic features of human papillomavirus-associated cervical disease. *Obstet. Gynecol. Clin. North Am.*, **20**, Mar;123-151

Reid, R., & Scalzi, P. (1985) Genital warts and cervical cancerVII. An improved colposcopic index for differentiating benign papillomaviral infections from high-grade cervical intraepithelial neoplasia. *Am. J. Obstet. Gynecol.*, **153**, 611-618

Richart, R.M. (1968) Natural history of cervical intraepithelial neoplasia. *Clin. Obstet. Gynecol.*, **5**, 748-784.

Richart, R.M. (1990) A modified terminology for cervical intraepithelial neoplasia. *Obstet. Gynecol.*, **75**, 131-133.

Sankaranarayanan, R., Black, R.J., & Parkin, D.M. (1998) *Cancer survival in developing countries*. IARC Scientific Publications No.145. International Agency for Research on Cancer, Lyon.

Sankaranarayanan, R., Wesley, R., Somanathan, T., Dhakad, N., Shyamalakumary, B., Sreedevi Amma, N., Parkin, D.M., & Krishnan Nair, M. (1998) Performance of visual inspection after acetic acid application (VIA) in the detection of cervical cancer precursors. *Cancer*, **83**, 2150-56

Sankaranarayanan, R., Budukh, A.M., & Rajkumar, R. (2001) Effective screening programmes for cervical cancer in low- and middle-income developing countries. *Bull. World Health. Organ.*, **79**, 954-62.

Schiffman, M.H., Brinton, L.A., Devesa, S.S., & Fraumeni, J.F. Jr. (1996) Cervical cancer. In: Schottenfeld, D., & Fraumeni, J.F., Jr (Eds). *Cancer epidemiology and prevention*. New York: Oxford University Press, 1090-116.

Schlecht, N.F., Kulaga, S., Robitaille, J., Ferreira, S., Santos, M., Miyamura, R.A., Duarte-Franco, E., Rohan, T.E., Ferenczy, A., Villa, L.L., & Franco, E.L. (2002) Persistent Human Papillomavirus Infection as a Predictor of Cervical Intraepithelial Neoplasia. *JAMA*, **286**, 3106-3114.

Sellors, J.W., Mahony, J.B., Kaczorowski, J., Lytwyn, A., Bangura, H., Chong, S., Lorincz, A., Dalby, D.M., Janjusevic, V., & Keller, J.L., for the Survey of HPV in Ontario Women (SHOW) Group. (2000) Prevalence and predictors of human papillomavirus infection in women in Ontario, Canada. *CMAJ*, **163**, 503-508.

Shafi, M.I., Luesley, D.M., Jordan, J.A., Dunn, J.A., Rollason, T.P., & Yates, M. (1997) Randomised trial of immediate versus deferred treatment strategies for the management of minor cervical cytological abnormalities. *Br. J. Obstet. Gynaecol*, **104**, 590-594.

Singer, A., & Monaghan, J. (2000) *Lower Genital Tract Precancer Colposcopy, Pathology and Treatment*. 2nd edition. Blackwell Science, Oxford.

Solomon, D. (1989) The 1988 Bethesda system for reporting cervical/vaginal cytologic diagnoses. Developed and approved at the National Cancer Institute Workshop, Bethesda, Maryland, USA, December, 12-13. *Acta. Cytol.*, **33**, 567-574.

Solomon, D., Davey, D., Kurman, R., Moriarty, A., O'Connor, D., Prey, M., Raab, S., Sherman, M., Wilbur, D., Wright Jr., T., & Young, N. (2002) The 2001 Bethesda system. Terminology for reporting results of cervical cytology. *JAMA*, **287**, 2114-2119.

Soutter, P. (1993) *Practical Colposcopy*. Oxford: Oxford University Press .

Stafl, A. & Wilbanks, G.D. (1991) An international terminology of colposcopy: Report of the nomenclature committee of the International Federation of Cervical Pathology and Colposcopy. *Obstet.Gynecol.*, **77**, 313-314

Thomas, G.M. (2000) Concurrent chemotherapy and radiation for locally advanced cervical cancer: the new standard of care. *Semin. Radiat. Oncol.*, **10**, 44-50

University of Zimbabwe/JHPIEGO Cervical Cancer Project. (1999) Visual inspection with acetic acid for cervical-cancer screening: test qualities in a primary-care setting. *Lancet*, **353**, 869-73.

Walboomers, J.M.M., Jacobs, M.V., Manos, M.M., Bosch, F.X., Kummer, J.A., Shah, K.V., Snijders, P.J., Peto, J., Meijer, C.J., & Munoz, N. (1999) Human papillomavirus is a necessary cause of invasive cervical cancer worldwide. *J. Pathol.*, **189**, 12-19.

Wallin, K.L., Wiklund, F., Ångström, T., Bergman, F., Stendahl, U., Wadell, G., Hallmans, G., & Dillner, J. (1999) Type-specific persistence of human papillomavirus DNA before the development of invasive cervical cancer. *N. Engl. J. Med.*, **341**, 1633-1638.

WHO guidelines for the management of sexually transmitted infections. http://www.who.int/HIVAIDS/STIcasemanagement/STIManagementguidelines/who_hiv_aids_2001.01/003.htm

William, J. (1888) *Cancer of the uterus: Harveian lectures for 1886*. HK Lewis, London.

Woodman CB, Collins S, Winter H, Bailey, A., Ellis, J., Prior, P., Yates, M., Rollason, T,P., & Young, L.S. (2001) Natural history of cervical human papillomavirus infection in young women: a longitudinal cohort study. *Lancet*, **357**, 1831-1836.

Wright, V.C., Lickrish, G.M., & Michael Shier, R. (1995) *Basic and Advanced Colposcopy. Part 1: A Practical Handbook for Treatment*, 2nd ed. Houston, Texas: Biomedical Communications.

Wright, V.C., Richart, M., & Ferenczy, A. (1992) Electrosurgery for HPV-related diseases of the lower genital tract. *A practical handbook for diagnosis and treatment by loop electrosurgical excision and fulguration procedures*. Arthur Vision, New York.

Wright, T.C. Jr, Subbarao, S., Ellerbrock, T.V., Lennox, J.L., Evans-Strickfaden, T., Smith, D.G., & Hart, C.E. (2001) Human immunodeficiency virus 1 expression in the female genital tract in association with cervical inflammation and ulceration. *Am. J. Obstet. Gynecol.*, **184**, 279-285.

Suggestions on further reading

ACCP. *Effectiveness, Safety and Acceptability of Cryotherapy: A Systematic Literature Review*. Seattle, Washington: PATH (2003).

Anderson M, Jordan J, Morse A, *et al. Integrated Colposcopy*. 2nd ed. London and New York: Chapman Hall Medical (1996).

Burghardt E, Pickel H, Girardi F. *Colposcopy Cervical Pathology. Textbook and Atlas*. Thieme, New York (1998).

Campion M, Ferris D, di Paola F, Reid R. *Modern colposcopy-A practical approach*. Augusta.Educational System Inc. 1991.

Cartier R, Cartier I. *Practical Colposcopy*. 3rd edition. Paris: Laboratoire Cartier (1993).

Coppleson M, Reid B, Pixley E. *Colposcopy*, 3rd Edition, Charles C Thomas, Springfield (1986).

Coppleson M, Dalrymple JC, Atkinson KH. Colposcopic differentiation of abnormalities arising in the transformation zone. *Obstetrics and Gynecology Clinics of North America* 20:83–110 (1993).

Franco E, Monsonego J. *New Developments in Cervical Cancer Screening and Prevention*. Oxford: Blackwell Science (1997).

IARC Monographs on the Evaluation of Carcinogenic Risks to Humans. Volume 64: Human Papillomaviruses. International Agency for Research on Cancer, Lyon (1995).

Singer A, Monaghan J. *Lower Genital Tract Precancer Colposcopy, Pathology and Treatment*. 2nd Edition. Blackwell Science, Oxford (2000).

Soutter P. *Practical Colposcopy*. Oxford: Oxford University Press (1993).

Wright VC, Lickrish GM, Shier RM. *Basic and Advanced Colposcopy*. Part 1: A Practical Handbook for Diagnosis, 2nd ed. Houston, Texas: Biomedical Communications (1995).

Wright VC, Lickrish GM, Shier RM. *Basic and Advanced Colposcopy*. Part 2: A Practical Handbook for Treatment, 2nd ed. Houston, Texas: Biomedical Communications (1995).

Wright TC, Richart RM, Ferenczy A. *Electrosurgery for HPV-related Diseases of the Lower Genital Tract*. New York, Arthur Vision Inc. (1992).

Appendix 1

Colposcopy record

1. Medical Record Number: _____

2. Patient's Name: _____

3. Age: _____

4. Date of visit: _____ / _____ / _____ (Day/Month/Year)

5. Colposcopist performing exam: _____

6. Did you see the entire squamocolumnar junction (SCJ)?   ❑ Yes   ❑ No

   (If 'No', consider endocervical curettage)

7. Unsatisfactory colposcopy: ❑ Entire SCJ not visualised   ❑ Entire lesion not visualised

8. Colposcopic findings within the transformation zone (use ✓ to indicate result):

   (Draw SCJ, acetowhite, punctation, mosaics, atypical vessels, and other lesions)

   ❑ Flat acetowhite epithelium

   ❑ Micropapillary or microconvoluted acetowhite epithelium

   ❑ Leukoplakia

   ❑ Punctation

   ❑ Mosaic

   ❑ Atypical vessels

   ❑ Iodine- negative epithelium

   ❑ Other, specify: _____

9. Findings outside the transformation zone: _____

   _____

10. Colposcopically suspect invasive carcinoma: Yes   No

11. Miscellaneous findings: _____

    _____

12. Colposcopic diagnosis (use ✓ to indicate result):

    ❑ Unsatisfactory, specify: _____

    ❑ Normal colposcopic findings

    ❑ Inflammation/infection, specify: _____

EXAMPLE

❑ Leukoplakia

❑ Condyloma

❑ Low-grade CIN

❑ High-grade CIN

❑ Invasive cancer, specify location of referral: _____

❑ Other, specify: _____

❑ Number of biopsies taken _____ (mark site(s) with an 'X' on colposcopy drawing)

❑ Endocervical curettage (ECC) taken

13. Other findings (use ✓ to indicate all that apply):

❑ Lesion extended into endocervix

❑ Mucosal bleeding easily induced

❑ Purulent cervicitis

❑ Opaque discharge

❑ Yellow discharge

❑ Other, specify: _____

14. Colposcopist's signature: _____

15. If test performed at colposcopy exam, note results below:

Cytology result:

❑ Negative

❑ Atypia/CIN 1

❑ CIN 2

❑ CIN 3

❑ Invasive cancer

ECC result:

❑ Negative

❑ CIN 1

❑ CIN 2

❑ CIN 3

❑ Microinvasive squamous cancer

❑ Invasive squamous cancer

❑ Adenocarcinoma

❑ Glandular dysplasia

❑ ECC not done

Biopsy result:

❑ Negative

❑ CIN 1

❑ CIN 2

❑ CIN 3

❑ Microinvasive squamous cancer

❑ Invasive squamous cancer

❑ Adenocarcinoma in-situ

❑ Adenocarcinoma

Patient's Name.............................   Health Center ....

Consent for Colposcopy, Biopsy, and Possible Treatment

Cervical cancer is a problem for women in our region, but much of it could be prevented by simple tests. The clinicians here are using a test that can find problems early. If these problems are found early, they can be treated easily and cancer can be avoided.

Procedures

You were referred for colposcopy because there is a possible problem with your cervix. If you decide to participate in this examination, the clinician will provide counselling and education about cervical cancer, ask you some questions about your reproductive history and risk of being pregnant, and examine your cervix today. S/he will use a speculum to hold the vagina open. Then, s/he will gently wipe your cervix with vinegar. You may feel a slight stinging from the vinegar. The clinician will look at your cervix with a colposcope, which magnifies and illuminates the cervix to help the clinician see your cervix more clearly. The colposcope will not touch your body. The examination will take about 5 to 7 minutes.

If the examination with the colposcope shows that your cervix is healthy, you will be finished with your examination. If the examination with the colposcope shows that your cervix is not healthy, the clinician will take a small sample of tissue from your cervix (this is called a biopsy) in order to check the diagnosis.

The biopsy may cause some pain that lasts a few seconds and varies from mild pinching to some cramping sensations. After the biopsy, you will be treated with cryotherapy to remove the area that is a problem on your cervix. You will probably feel some cramping during and after the procedure; the cramping usually stops shortly after the procedure. You also will probably experience spotting or light bleeding from your cervix for 1 to 2 weeks and a watery vaginal discharge that lasts 2 to 4 weeks. You will be asked to not have sexual intercourse for 3 to 4 weeks to allow your cervix to heal properly. You also will be asked to return to the clinic 9-12 months after the procedure for a follow-up visit. The clinician will look at your cervix again with a colposcope in order to make sure that the treatment was successful. If, however, the colposcopic examination shows that the treatment was not successful, you will be advised on further steps to take.

Risks

You may be embarrassed by the vaginal examination. The colposcopy examination may cause vaginal irritation and burning for several minutes. You may experience slight vaginal bleeding for one or two days if a biopsy is taken from your cervix. You may experience a watery vaginal discharge for up to four weeks if you undergo treatment by cryotherapy. Although it is unlikely, you also may experience heavy vaginal bleeding. There is a 10% risk that cryotherapy, if used correctly, will not be effective, but this outcome will be detected at the follow-up examination after 9-12 months.

Eligibility

Before being examined, you will be asked a series of questions to determine if there is a chance of your being pregnant. If so, you will be tested with a standard urine pregnancy test. You will be examined using colposcopy regardless of your pregnancy status. If you require treatment and the pregnancy test is positive, your treatment will be postponed until six weeks after delivery.

Confidentiality

All of your personal information will be kept confidential and used only for your medical care. Any other use will require your written consent. If you refuse any part of this examination, it will not affect care that we give you in the future.

Questions

Please direct any questions you have about the examination or your rights as a patient to district hospital staff.

Patient Statement (Provider's copy)

The information above on colposcopy, biopsy, and possible treatment has been explained to me and I have been given the opportunity to ask questions. I agree to participate in this examination.

_____

Signature of patient   OR   thumbprint of patient ➔

Date _____

_____

Signature of witness

Date _____

- -

(tear off at dotted line and give to patient)

Patient Statement (Patient's copy)

The information above on colposcopy, biopsy, and possible treatment has been explained to me and I have been given the opportunity to ask questions. I agree to participate in this examination.

_____

Signature of patient   OR   thumbprint of patient ➔

Date _____

_____

Signature of witness

Date _____

Preparation of 5% acetic acid, Lugol's iodine solution, and Monsel's paste

5% dilute acetic acid

Ingredients	Quantity
1. Glacial acetic acid	5 ml
2. Distilled water	95 ml

Preparation
Carefully add 5 ml of glacial acetic acid into 95 ml of distilled water and mix thoroughly.

Storage:
Unused acetic acid should be discarded at the end of the day.

Label:
5% dilute acetic acid

Note: It is important to remember to dilute the glacial acetic acid, since the undiluted strength causes a severe chemical burn if applied to the epithelium.

Lugol's iodine solution

Ingredients	Quantity
1. Potassium iodide	10 g
2. Distilled water	100 ml
3. Iodine crystals	5 g

Preparation
A. Dissolve 10 g potassium iodide in 100 ml of distilled water.
B. Slowly add 5 g iodine crystals, while shaking.
C. Filter and store in a tightly stoppered brown bottle.

Storage:
1 month

Label:
Lugol's iodine solution
Use by (date)

Monsel's paste

Ingredients	Quantity
1. Ferric sulfate base	15 g
2. Ferrous sulfate powder	a few grains
3. Sterile water for mixing	10 ml
4. Glycerol starch (see preparation on next page)	12 g

Preparation

Take care: The reaction is exothermic (emits heat).
A. Add a few grains of ferrous sulfate powder to 10 ml of sterile water in a glass beaker. Shake.
B. Dissolve the ferric sulfate base in the solution by stirring with a glass stick. The solution should become crystal clear.
C. Weigh the glycerol starch in a glass mortar. Mix well.
D. Slowly add ferric sulfate solution to glycerol starch, constantly mixing to get a homogeneous mixture.
E. Place in a 25 ml brown glass bottle.
F. For clinical use, most clinics prefer to allow enough evaporation to give the solution a sticky pastelike consistency that looks like mustard. This may take 2 to 3 weeks, depending on the environment. The top of the container can then be secured for storage. If necessary, sterile water can be added to the paste to thin it.
Note: This preparation contains 15% elementary iron.

Storage:
6 months

Label:
Monsel's solution
Shake well
External use only
Use by (date)

Glycerol starch
(an ingredient in Monsel's paste)

Ingredients	Quantity
1. Starch	30 g
2. Sterile water for mixing	30 ml
3. Glycerine	390 g

Preparation

A. In a china crucible, dissolve the starch in the sterile water.
B. Add the glycerine. Shake well.
C. Heat the crucible and its contents over a bunsen burner. Mix constantly with a spatula until the mass takes on a thick, swelling consistency. Take care not to overheat so as not to let it turn yellow.

Storage:
1 year

Label:
Glycerol starch
Store in a cool place
For external use only
Use by (date)
Note: Do not overheat, otherwise the mixture will turn yellow.

Colposcopic terminology

Normal colposcopic findings

Original squamous epithelium
Columnar epithelium
Normal transformation zone

Abnormal colposcopic findings

Within the transformation zone
    Acetowhite epithelium
        Flat
        Micropapillary or microconvoluted
    Punctation*
    Mosaic*
    Leukoplakia*
    Iodine-negative epithelium
    Atypical vessels
Outside the transformation zone, e.g., ectocervix, vagina
    Acetowhite epithelium*
        Flat
        Micropapillary or microconvoluted
    Punctation*
    Mosaic*
    Leukoplakia*

    Iodine-negative epithelium
    Atypical vessels
Colposcopically suspect invasive carcinoma
Unsatisfactory colposcopy
    Squamocolumnar junction not visible
    Severe inflammation or severe atrophy
    Cervix not visible
Miscellaneous findings
    Nonacetowhite micropapillary surface
    Exophytic condyloma
    Inflammation
    Atrophy
    Ulcer
    Other

*   Indicates minor or major change. Minor changes are acetowhite epithelium, fine mosaic, fine punctation, and thin leukoplakia. Major changes are dense acetowhite epithelium, coarse mosaic, coarse punctation, thick leukoplakia, atypical vessels, and erosion.

Ref: Stafl and Wilbanks (1991)

The modified Reid colposcopic index (RCI)*

The modified Reid colposcopic index (RCI)*			
Colposcopic signs	Zero point	One point	Two points
Colour	Low-intensity acetowhitening (not completely opaque); indistinct acetowhitening; transparent or translucent acetowhitening Acetowhitening beyond the margin of the transformation zone Pure snow-white colour with intense surface shine (rare)	Intermediate shade - grey/white colour and shiny surface (most lesions should be scored in this category)	Dull, opaque, oyster white; grey
Lesion margin and surface configuration	Microcondylomatous or micropapillary contour[1] Flat lesions with indistinct margins Feathered or finely scalloped margins Angular, jagged lesions[3] Satellite lesions beyond the margin of the transformation zone	Regular-shaped, symmetrical lesions with smooth, straight outlines	Rolled, peeling edges[2] Internal demarcations between areas of differing colposcopic appearance—a central area of high-grade change and peripheral area of low-grade change
Vessels	Fine/uniform-calibre vessels[4]- closely and uniformly placed Poorly formed patterns of fine punctation and/or mosaic Vessels beyond the margin of the transformation zone Fine vessels within microcondylomatous or micropapillary lesions[6]	Absent vessels	Well defined coarse punctation or mosaic, sharply demarcated[5] - and randomly and widely placed

The modified Reid colposcopic index (RCI)*(Cont.)

Colposcopic signs	Zero point	One point	Two points
Iodine staining	Positive iodine uptake giving mahogany-brown color Negative uptake of insignificant lesion, i.e., yellow staining by a lesion scoring three points or less on the first three criteria Areas beyond the margin of the transformation zone, conspicuous on colposcopy, evident as iodine-negative areas (such areas are frequently due to parakeratosis)[7]	Partial iodine uptake - variegated, speckled appearance	Negative iodine uptake of significant lesion, i.e., yellow staining by a lesion already scoring four points or more on the first three criteria

* Colposcopic grading performed with 5% aqueous acetic acid and Lugol's iodine solution. (See Appendix 3 for recipes for 5% acetic acid and for Lugol's iodine solution).

1 Microexophytic surface contour indicative of colposcopically overt cancer is not included in this scheme.

2 Epithelial edges tend to detach from underlying stroma and curl back on themselves. Note: Prominent low-grade lesions often are overinterpreted, while subtle avascular patches of HSIL can easily be overlooked.

3 Score zero even if part of the peripheral margin does have a straight course.

4 At times, mosaic patterns containing central vessels are characteristic of low-grade histological abnormalities. These low-grade-lesion capillary patterns can be quite pronounced. Until the physician can differentiate fine vascular patterns from coarse, overdiagnosis is the rule.

5 Branching atypical vessels indicative of colposcopically overt cancer are not included in this scheme.

6 Generally, the more microcondylomatous the lesion, the lower the score. However, cancer also can present as a condyloma, although this is a rare occurrence.

7 Parakeratosis: a superficial zone of cornified cells with retained nuclei.

Colposcopic prediction of histologic diagnosis using the Reid Colposcopic Index (RCI)

RCI (overall score)	Histology
0 – 2	Likely to be CIN 1
3 – 4	Overlapping lesion: likely to be CIN 1 or CIN 2
5 – 8	Likely to be CIN 2-3

Index

Acetowhitening 35, 59-65, 70, 81, 87, 128

Adenocarcinoma 19, 23, 72

Adenocarcinoma *in situ* 13, 19, 72

Adenosquamous carcinoma 24

Anal intraepithelial neoplasia (AIN) 36

Atypical squamous cells of undetermined significance (ASCUS) 14-15

Atypical surface vessels 70-74

Atypical transformation zone (ATZ) 11-12, 41

Bethesda system 14-15

Blended cutting waveform 104

Branching surface vessels 47, 48

Carcinoma *in situ* (CIS) 13, 14

Cervical intraepithelial neoplasia (CIN) 13-19, 55-68, 95-111

Cervical stenosis 102, 111

Cervicitis 79

Cervicovaginitis 79

Coagulation waveform 104

Coarse mosaic 57-58, 67, 87, 128

Coarse punctation 58, 63, 87, 128

Cold-knife conization 43, 92, 93, 110

Colposcope 29, 31

Colposcopic terminology 127

Colposcopy record 29, 36, 121

Columnar epithelium 4-5, 48, 49, 53

Condyloma 14, 58, 92

Congenital transformation zone 12, 53

Consent form 38, 123

Cryotherapy (cryo) 89, 95-102

Crypts 5, 10

Decontamination 113-116

Dysplasia 13-15

Ectocervix 1-3

Ectopy 7, 8

Ectropion 7, 8

Endocervix 2, 3

Endocervical curettage (ECC) 42-43

Fine mosaic 58, 67, 87, 128

Fine puncuation 58, 67, 87, 128

Fulguration 104, 107

Glandular dysplasia 93

High-grade squamous intraepithelial lesion (HSIL) 14-15

High-level disinfection 113-116

Histopathology 16, 24

Hyperkeratosis 30, 58, 92

Hyperplasia 8

Immature metaplasia 9-10, 50-54

International Federation of Gynaecology and Obstetrics (FIGO) staging system 24-25

Inflammatory lesions 64, 79-83

Keratinizing squamous cell carcinoma 23-24

Leopard skin appearance 82

Leukoplakia 30, 58, 86, 92

Loop electrosurgical excision procedure (LEEP) 103-111

Low-grade squamous intraepithelial lesion (LSIL) 14-15

Lugol's iodine solution 36, 41, 51, 65, 81, 125

Mature squamous metaplasia 9-12, 36, 51, 87

Microinvasive carcinoma 21-27

Monsel's paste 42, 126

Nabothian cyst/follicle 10

New squamocolumnar junction 5-8

Non-keratinizing squamous cell carcinoma 24

Pregnancy 43-44, 93-94

Reid Colposcopic Index 128

Reproductive tract infection 91-92

Schiller's test (see also Lugol's iodine solution) 36

Squamocolumnar junction (SCJ) 5-8, 87

Squamous metaplasia 8-11, 50-51

Sterilization 113-116

Stratified non-keratinizing squamous epithelium 3-4

Transformation zone (TZ) 11-12, 53-54, 67, 87

Umbilication 58

Vaginal intraepithelial neoplasia (VAIN) 36

Visual inspection with acetic acid (VIA) 29-36, 41, 49, 59-65, 81, 87, 125

Visual inspection with acetic acid using magnification (VIAM) 29-36

Vulvar intraepithelial neoplasia (VIN) 36